Mindful Leadership: A Guide for the Health Care Professions

Mindful Leadership

A Guide for the Health Care Professions

CHRISTOPHER JOHNS

 palgrave

First published 2016 by
PALGRAVE

Palgrave in the UK is an imprint of Macmillan Publishers Limited, registered in England, company number 785998, of 4 Crinan Street, London, N1 9XW.

Palgrave Macmillan in the US is a division of St Martin's Press LLC, 175 Fifth Avenue, New York, NY 10010.

Palgrave is the global imprint of the above companies and is represented throughout the world.

Palgrave® and Macmillan® are registered trademarks in the United States, the United Kingdom, Europe and other countries.

ISBN 978–1–137–54099–7 paperback

This book is printed on paper suitable for recycling and made from fully managed and sustained forest sources. Logging, pulping and manufacturing processes are expected to conform to the environmental regulations of the country of origin.

A catalogue record for this book is available from the British Library.

A catalog record for this book is available from the Library of Congress.

Printed in China

Contents

List of Tables and Figures

Tables

Figures

Preface

Nothing ever becomes real until it is experienced

John Keats[1]

This book is about becoming a mindful leader. As Wheatley and Kellner-Rogers (1998: 88) write, 'Life is in perpetual motion, "becoming, becoming". The motions of life swirl inward to the creating of self and outward to the creating of the world. We turn inward to bring forth a self. Then the self extends outwards, seeking other, joining together.'

Becoming a leader is vital because leadership is the hub that drives health care, and leadership is sorely lacking. In the UK, over the past ten years, successive government white papers have called for a dynamic leadership to take forward health care reforms. In a circular to NHS trusts in October 2009 concerned with the latest quality initiative, the NHS Chief Executive, David Nicholson, stated the need for the *right focus of leadership* and *right leadership* (Department of Health 2009a). Whilst Nicholson recognised the need, he did not set out a vision for leadership beyond indicating that it was essentially concerned with ensuring quality and service delivery – a somewhat narrow and functional approach. Whilst ensuring quality of service delivery is clearly an important leadership task, it is something a leader does, it is not essentially about who a leader is.

Leadership is essentially concerned with relationships rather than outcomes, although this is not to diminish the significance of outcomes, especially within a health care culture that has become fixated on targets and outcomes. However, get the process right, and the right outcomes will be achieved with greater quality, productivity and satisfaction.

Leadership is the organisation's life spirit. When it glows brightly, people buzz with creativity, enthusiasm and goodwill in common purpose. Without leadership, organisations stumble in darkness. So ask yourself, 'Why has cultivating leadership within health care been so limited?' It seems there is a three-fold erroneous assumption that: first, practitioners have skills of leadership; second, the nature of leadership is misunderstood; and third, leadership already exists. As such, leadership is a rare quality within the transactional culture of NHS organisations with its mantra of command and control. Hence, aspiring leaders in health care are uncertain about what it is to be a leader because they rarely experience leadership.

Because of its culture, the transactional organisation cannot accommodate leadership, at least on any real level. In fact, these organisations naturally resist leadership because it threatens its own learnt cultural patterns of working that govern it. As such, there exists a tension between the idea of leadership and its lived reality. Understanding and working towards resolving this tension forms the basis for becoming a leader, as I shall expand on through the text. It is this tension I invite the reader to dialogue with, flow with and hopefully grow with.

Everybody has the potential to be a leader, no matter what his or her practice discipline or role within the organisation. I have noted the danger of assuming that practitioners have the skills of leadership (Alimo-Metcalfe 2002). Bennett and Robinson (2003) agree, highlighting that organisations and educationalists make too many assumptions about the existing leadership knowledge and skills of clinicians. These authors argue that changing personal values, beliefs and attitudes is as important as knowledge and skills development to fit practitioners for their expanding role. If these changes are to be integrated with theoretical and practical knowledge, then it has to be recognised that learning about leadership is impossible to separate from learning about self.

When I think of great leaders I am immediately drawn to Nelson Mandela. I say this not from sentimentality considering his recent passing (November 2013), but simply because of his immense presence across the world stage. He said, 'It is better to lead from behind and to put others in front, especially when you celebrate victory when nice things occur. You take the front line when there is danger. Then people will appreciate your leadership.'[2] These words suggest a leadership that works behind the scenes creating an environment for achievement. When necessary, it steps forward to take the lead so people feel secure.

Living in Cornwall I was amused by a beer mat showing a picture of Nelson Mandela waving with a pasty in his hand quoting – 'A good head, a good heart and a good pasty are always a formidable combination.'[3] Put another way, leaders must appropriately feed their good heads and good hearts. Pasties sustained Cornish miners in their hard work for centuries! This book is akin to a Cornish pasty to sustain leaders as they mine at becoming leaders.

My interest in leadership evolved from my position as general manager at Burford Community Hospital when I inquired into my role as clinical leader

of a hospital practising primary nursing team. My own leadership development had been non-existent. I had once attended a first line management
course. Note that it was a management course, not a leadership course.
Perhaps leadership is considered innate or simply learnt through diffusion
when exposed long enough to practice. As Porter-O'Grady (1992: 18) suggests, 'most leaders have no leadership training and that they learnt on the
job'. Surely, any organisation that values its human resource would invest
in its staff to bring out their best performance? Given the human resource
cost it doesn't make sense not to. Issues of best performance are inextri-
cably linked to issues of quality and clinical governance. The Department
of Health (1998) in their white paper A First Class Service defined clinical
governance as 'a framework through which organisations are accountable
for continually improving the quality of their services and safeguarding high
standards of care by creating an environment in which excellence in clinical
care can flourish'. To flourish is to grow or develop in a healthy or vigor-
ous way (Chambers 2005: 385). Perhaps they should have stated 'in which
practitioners can flourish'. This sends out a different message – a focus on
people rather than outcomes.

Jaworski (1998: 66) notes, 'leadership is all about the release of human
possibilities'. These words capture something of the greatness of leadership and its moral endeavour. Such words inspire me as I seek to realise
leadership in my own practice, whether as an educationalist or as a therapist working with patients in a hospice. It doesn't matter whether I manage
people or not. What matters is that I am part of a team and take responsibility for leading myself as part of that team working collaboratively towards
realising a shared vision.

Structure of the book

The book is arranged to draw you into new ways of seeing leadership. It
is grounded in the narratives of aspiring leaders as part of a collaborative
inquiry into becoming a leader. Each leader agreed to make their narrative
available for analysis and possible publication. More than eighty narratives
have been constructed, offering a rich source of data to develop my insights
on realising leadership within NHS organisations across various disciplines.
Only six of these narratives were constructed by men. I sense this reflects
that leadership is generally viewed as soft and feminine in contrast with management, which is viewed as hard and masculine. This makes sense when one
considers the patriarchal nature of society. The narratives are compelling
as they reveal the leaders' struggles to overcome barriers, both embodied
within self and embedded in normal patterns of organisational relationships,

towards realising desirable leadership. No matter the discipline the song remains the same although to varying degrees. The transactional organisation emerges as a machine with rigid systems that seeks to maintain its own flawed smooth running. In such environments, humanness is diminished. It is a place without soul, constrained by its own systems, a place of alienation from self and others that stands in ironic and perverse contrast with the mandate of health care organisations to care. Yet, in spite of itself, the transactional organisation does not run smoothly. We know because the press continue to report situations of poor patient care and low staff morale. The *West Briton* headlined just this week (Thursday 12 March 2015), 'Morale at RCHT is still getting worse'. It reports (see figure below) 'Overworked, under pressure and convinced their work makes no difference – that's how thousands of NHS staff in Cornwall feel about their jobs, according to an annual health check on morale in the workforce.'

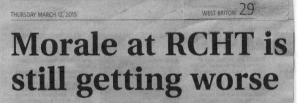

The survey report is a devastating failure of leadership. RCHT displays the label 'Investors in People', but you must wonder what that means in the face of such low staff morale. But it needn't be like that. We can have healthy care organisations whose primary function is to facilitate leadership so staff are in the best shape to respond to the core business of effective patient care. It is not difficult to appreciate that people who are valued, given responsibility and feel cared for will be more productive and satisfied. Patients and families would get better care. The two things are reciprocal. Morale would be sky high.

In 'Visions of Leadership' (Chapter 1) I introduce the idea of being mindful or mindfulness that underlines leadership, no matter what adjective precedes it. Mindfulness is the culmination of dedicated reflective practice over time. I then explore some ideas of leadership, yet I am not overly concerned with leadership theory or current initiatives in leadership development within the NHS. These are easily appreciated through a Google search. Indeed, any leader serious about becoming a leader will investigate and consider these leadership ideas in terms of their personal leadership development. As such, the book is not a treatise on the nature of leadership although ideas of leadership are in constant dialogue with the aspiring leaders' collective and individual narratives. However, I do draw on some ideas from leadership theory and leadership development as appropriate. These are often located within the narratives where they can be considered from a contextual perspective. The focus on transformational leadership reflects the rhetoric that transformational leadership is the model for health care leadership in contrast with a transactional type leadership that characterises health care organisations. Of increasing relevance is the emergence of servant leadership as a leadership approach that radically shifts the nature of power within organisational relationships. Prosser (2010) notes that servant leadership is more of a philosophy of leadership than a theory of leadership. I explore the significance of leadership as feminine, as caring and as chaotic, and in doing so add contrast to the idea of leadership as something broader and more philosophical than the narrower idea of particular theories. Ideas about leadership should not be viewed as prescriptive but simply as ideas to help the emerging leader formulate his or her own vision of leadership. As such, I offer my own vision of leadership as an exemplar of constructing a bespoke vision emerging from the influence of servant leadership.

Words are one thing, but living those words congruently is quite another, especially in a health care organisational culture that is inherently transactional. Indeed, the transactional culture may resist the emergence of true leadership because this threatens the norms that govern it, in particular the way relationships are governed by power. The power of norms or culture cannot be underestimated as ideas of leadership are inevitably distorted to fit in within existing norms. So whilst most health care organisations espouse the idea of leadership few achieve it in any meaningful way. The leader must become aware of the way these norms pattern his or her relationships within the organisation. This requires seeing self objectively, becoming mindful of self and appreciating the way one's thinking, feeling and behaviour is influenced by such norms. In this process of understanding, the leader becomes increasingly mindful of the tension between realising leadership within the transactional organisation. This raises an obvious question – how will I know if I am responding in tune with my leadership values? To reiterate, the key is reflection – the leader's ability to reflect on his or her leadership performance in such a way as to see clearly the tension between desirable leadership practice and the way he or she actually practises. In doing so, those forces that constrain leadership will be identified, understood and, over time, shifted within a reflexive developmental spiral. I show some results of scanning the web for ideas on leadership and finally note NHS leadership development within the UK, notably the Leadership Academy model. This reference is brief because any leader who is interested can easily access this information via the web.

'The Adventure Has Only Just Begun' (Chapter 2) is Martha's narrative of becoming a transformational leader. It gives the reader insight into her leadership journey over twenty-eight months. The narrative starkly reveals her effort to understand and work towards resolving the creative tension between her transformational vision and the transactional nature of the organisation in which she works. Her understanding of the transactional organisation is vital because she had never considered its nature before. She had simply taken it for granted. As she begins to understand it so she can begin to liberate herself from its shackles even as it resists and obstructs her through its pattern of relationships and systems.

She initially had no more than a theoretical idea of leadership gleaned largely from the leadership literature. She adopts a transformational vision using Schuster's attributes. Her effort emerges as emotional and frustrating, but ultimately joyful, as she breaks through the barriers that constrained realising her vision. She has a remarkable ability to see things clearly, almost dispassionately. The apparent ease of her transition into transformational leadership masks a steely determination and deep passion. She illustrates what can be achieved against the odds with her vision, her determination and a genuine sense of caring.

In 'The Learning Organisation' (Chapter 3) I posit creating and sustaining the learning organisation as the primary task of leadership, where people, both individually and collectively, can dialogue and grow. Martha referred to this development in her narrative. The learning organisation is inspired by the work of Senge (1990) who sets out its five disciplines. Perhaps if clinical governance was viewed through such a dynamic lens, then approaches to quality and performance would be radically different with every staff person becoming actively involved. Leadership is always concerned with establishing the conditions of 'living quality' rather than viewing quality as something imposed. I posit leadership as a sixth discipline it being the power that drives the learning organisation. Significant ideas such as community and dialogue are explored within the disciplines.

'It's Automatic, Isn't It?'(Chapter 4) unfolds Alison's narrative of becoming a servant leader. Alison is the manager of a psychiatric unit for the elderly. Her narrative shares many similarities with Martha's narrative in Chapter 2 in their struggle to realise leadership from within the transactional organisation. Alison offers insight into conflict modes of response, highlighting that conflict can be harnessed as a positive energy for change, reflecting two things that leaders need to do effectively. Conflict and change are in many ways symbiotic in that change always surfaces conflict in its challenge to the status quo and in that conflict is always an opportunity for learning and change. Conflict and change are both dynamic ways of being yet they are often imbued with a negative sense. As Skjorshammer (2002: 915) notes, 'A major challenge in professional cooperation is managing disagreements and conflicts ... is an important determinant of quality of care and effectiveness in a hospital setting.' I would add that managing conflict skilfully is the major challenge of organisational life. Conflict by its nature is emotionally charged leaving people exhausted and drained.

Through guiding emerging leaders, I know that conflict is an everyday event. The root of conflict can lie anywhere, often triggered by unresolved underlying issues caused by poor communication, divergent values and agendas, power differentials, ego and personality, injustice, rivalry, lack of respect and support, and perhaps most of all lack of leadership. Conflict is perhaps the most difficult situation for people. One reason is its strong emotional connection. In reply, the most common response to conflict is avoidance. This is perhaps more so for nurses caught in the caring compassion trap (Dickson 1982) where surfacing issues of conflict may seem the antithesis of caring. Responding to conflict may breech the 'harmonious team' that demands loyalty to the team even to the detriment of patient care (Johns 2009). The harmonious team is a social defence system against anxiety or, put more colloquially, a form of social etiquette. Osho (1994: 59) poses the question 'Why does society need etiquette?' He replies, 'Because everybody is so violent. If there was no etiquette, we would be at each other's throats continuously.'

Hence, to breech etiquette would be to evoke violence. Perhaps people think it better to brush the conflict under the carpet and pretend that nothing has happened. Yet conflict does not go away. It leaves a trace and festers. It accumulates and manifests itself in stressful behaviour. It leaks out in indirect ways causing more conflict and creating toxic environments that are harmful rather than healing. Yet conflict for the leader can be turned around and viewed as a positive event, an opportunity for learning. Modes of responding to conflict can be appreciated through using Thomas and Kilmann's conflict mode instrument (1974).

In 'Leading Change, Easing Conflict' (Chapter 5) I reflect on my own leadership history. Although I was not fully aware at the time, my leadership was pivotal to developing clinical practice and quality at these hospitals. Fundamental to this work was change and with it conflict management. The leader by nature is always curious about practice, always asking the question, 'How can care be developed more effectively in terms of patient processes and outcomes?' Of course change impacts on the status quo and creates conflict. Yet within the learning organisation, conflict is itself a motivating factor towards change. I explore models for both change and conflict management.

'No One Said This Would Be Easy' (Chapter 6) is Pia's narrative of becoming a leader. The narrative offers deep insights into the way the transactional organisation can oppress its staff due to high anxiety and patterns of managing anxiety based on authoritative power and parent–child patterns of relating. Her narrative reflects the typical struggle that leaders faced in their effort to realise leadership as something lived within their transactional health care organisations. I say typical because all the leadership narratives portray this same compelling message – that the transactional organisation will always resist true leadership, despite rhetoric to the contrary, in its effort to maintain the status quo. This resistance is not a conscious act of resistance. It is fine wired within its systems. The emerging leaders themselves are also fine wired. Therefore, in order to become a leader they must firstly appreciate and secondly resolve the tension between an understanding of their current reality and their vision of leadership. It is the creative learning moment. Pia's particular struggle is revealed in a pattern of oppression within her relationships with two managers, both women, both midwives in middle management positions. These managers are anxious and brittle. In their efforts to control their environment they respond to their anxiety through characteristic authoritative power and parent–child patterns of relating. Time and time again Pia is knocked back just when things seem to be easing. Yet she perseveres. It is a narrative of empowerment. She questions whether the effort was worth it. The transactional environment is revealed as a joyless and toxic place to be, a place where, entangled in the transactional systems where everyone has become an object, people have lost sight of caring. It is a moral wasteland where love and caring withers and perishes.

'The Road to Oz' (Chapter 7) is Lisa's journey of becoming a leader. She constructs a puzzle of unravelling old ways of being as a foundation for constructing a new leadership way of being. It is a significant story because it reveals that the journey of becoming a leader is complex It isn't simply a cognitive idea but a deeper ontological journey whereby the leader has to go deep inside and find herself in order to change herself. This takes time and guidance. Whilst initiatives such as the modern matron appear on the surface to be an attempt to recover a sense of leadership, it is more an attempt to recover a sense of order battered by complaints of poor care and infection.

I coined the metaphor 'The Bubble in the Machine' (Chapter 8) to symbolise the way leadership can be insidiously accommodated within the transactional system. Without doubt, all the leaders realised their visions of leadership to some extent. In doing so, they created these bubbles as subversive movements that shift the organisation from within, without apparently altering its surface pyramidal shape. The transactional world does not easily accommodate a transformational leadership even though it espouses leadership as desirable. This says something about the way leadership is conceptually viewed and valued.

I reveal and explore the tension in realising leadership within the transactional organisation. What emerges is a profound difference between these two approaches and the realisation that there is no smooth continuum from one to the other simply because there is real dichotomy. They are fundamentally different and probably incompatible ways of being in the world. This is why the transactional must resist the transformational because it disrupts normal patterns of relating based on tradition, authority and embodiment. Ideas such as power and transactional analysis are explored to frame these social norms.

If health care organisations want genuine leadership then they must seriously invest in leader development through sustained and skilful group coaching based on a vision of leadership as suggested through this book, rather than on a narrow focus on managing quality and driving through change like puppets reacting to imposed demand. I argue this approach should be throughout the whole organisation from top to bottom. The whole organisation needs to be engaged and working together to transform itself into a vibrant mindful leadership milieu to ensure the most effective care and a fulfilled workforce.

Appendix A1 sets out the MSc Health Care Leadership programme at the University of Bedfordshire. Appendix A2 outlines reflexive narrative as a journey of self-inquiry and transformation towards realising a vision of leadership as a lived reality.

Throughout the book I refer to aspiring leaders. As the vast majority of these leaders are women (92 percent) I usually use the female pronoun. Where I do use 'he' it is in relation to the fact that I refer to a male aspiring leader.[4]

As narratives are revealing, I have changed names and locations. The narratives are statements of professional responsibility that reflect the leader's endeavour to become a desired leader towards creating better health care practice. Yet the ethical will always be controversial in a transactional culture that fails to tolerate any criticism of its practice, even when that criticism leads to more effective health care.

I have written the book as a reflective text to open a dialogical space to trigger the reader's engagement and reflection on her own leadership. To engage is to be open to the possibilities of what the text has to say, to keep an open mind and to be aware of your assumptions and prejudices. Do not take offence. Nothing I have written is intended to be authoritative. It is, of course, the way a mindful leader would approach any text.

Hannah writes:

> I invite my readers to ride in tandem with me viewing the moving scenery through the filter of their own experience and applying it to their own lives. I depend on you, the reader, to move the narrative beyond an articulation of personal experience into the realm of wider interpretation and social relevance (Pinar 1981). It is from you that the text gains its validity and movement. Stories can infect perceptions, invade complacency, amplify conscience and change lives. Stories are living things and their real life begins when they start to live in you (Okri 1997: 44).

> I would like to take this opportunity to thank Otter, my wife and inspiration, all my MSc leadership in health care students 2002-2014 without whose collaboration this book would not have been possible, and Palgrave for having faith.

Notes

1. www.brainyquotes
2. Mandela N. (no date) (online) Available from www.dictionary.com (Accessed 8 January 2005).
3. www.cornish.co.uk
4. A narrative written by a male emerging leader has been published – 'More than Eggs for Breakfast' in *Guided reflection: A narrative approach to advancing practice* (2010) edited by C. Johns. Exemplars of leadership around issues of chaos and change written by aspiring leaders in assignments have been published in *Becoming a reflective practitioner*, 4th edition (2013) by C. Johns.

Foreword

Today, if one is fully present and listens from the heart, one can feel the deep sense of longing in health care. It is as if millions of voices are crying out for a sense of hope and direction amidst the chaos of the rising patient acuity, the churn of turnover, the challenges of reimbursement, the focus on the bottom line and the declining health and disengagement of the workforce. There is a longing for leadership that creates a path back to that sense of meaning and impact – that connection with our deepest human purpose that brings out the best in us and unites us all in a common mission. There is a longing for caring leaders who bring clarity of voice and moments of peace and joy to environments of turbulence, constant change, fire fighting and adrenalin addiction – a strong and true voice that removes the obstacles, confronts issues, frames conflict, protects the vulnerable, attracts and grows talent and builds the infrastructure for exemplary professional practice within a healthy work environment. Leaders who relate to humanity in a wiser and more compassionate way are essential to our survival.

The first step to becoming a leader is knowledge of self. Knowledge of self is not possible without continuous, disciplined reflection. The willingness to take this joyful and painful learning journey into awareness and then knowledge of self takes courage and guidance. In this book, Johns has illustrated practitioners in their daily interactions mindfully striving to evolve as leaders. In their voices, one hears joy, pain, struggle and discovery. By creating structured reflection and integrating the components of transformational leadership, we witness in this book how development of leaders can be accelerated. As practitioners grow in understanding of self through reflection, they are able to take the next step in evolution as a leader, that of attunement with others. Leadership becomes possible through relationships. Leadership is all about our ability to influence through those relationships. Relationships are not possible without respect and the empathy found in attunement.

Leaders are paradoxes. They are artists who manage the creative tension of what is right, along with the dance of politics and the focus on the bottom line. They can be gentle and compassionate, yet fearless, tough and persistent warriors. Leaders are steel within a velvet glove. They are about setting high standards, developing others and holding them close with feedback, and then letting go. They are humble yet confident risk takers. They are about balance yet realise that the status quo is not an option. They constantly practise reflection and are continuously learning.

Leaders create a safe space, an ecosystem within systems, a subculture within a culture where people thrive and actualise their fullest potential. This safe space can be found in minute-to-minute interactions when fully awakened leaders use every opportunity, and in the micro-intimate, mindful moments of being totally present, and used to connect with individuals and take actions that lead to a goal, never missing an opportunity. Many of these interactions are illustrated in the journaling of Johns' practitioners.

Leaders are lighthouses, beacons in the perfect storm of health care, shining the light on issues, identifying talent, clarifying the right thing to do, bringing out the best in others and creating a shared vision and path to follow. Because of their light, consistent moral compass and authentic style, they attract followers and inspire hope. In order for health care to find its way back to its purpose, transformational leaders must be present at all levels of organisational life, from senior administration where the patient becomes visible through the voice of a practitioner at the table in the boardroom, to the point of care, where a skilfully engaged practitioner gives of mind, heart, hand and spirit in every interchange. The purpose of health care is to create healing environments where patients, families and practitioners team up to learn from one another and support one another through the joys and challenges of the human experience and thus become intertwined with our journey through life.

Becoming a leader, no matter what adjective we place before it – whether reflective, servant or transformational – requires a courageous willingness to dig deep and discover our authentic self, a commitment to serve, to be present in the dialogue of everyday life, to seek feedback and be willing to continuously grow by constantly stopping to notice and digest what is happening around us. Leaders have an innate sense of generativity – the passion to grow and develop others. As the reader experiences the voices of the practitioners in this book, one feels the discomfort of growth as they stretch out of their comfort zone with a driving passion to grow.

Reading this book, a beautiful tapestry of the voices of practitioners interwoven with analysis and supported by the literature on leadership, provides a contemplative opportunity to renew and redirect the 'learning reader'. Learning means 'change in behaviour', and if perhaps a passage strikes a chord and if we all take but one thing from this book and evolve our practice, we as a community of nurses have made a commitment to change the landscape of health care across the globe.

Pamela Klauer Triolo
Chief Nursing Officer, UPMC
Associate Dean, Academic-Service Partnerships
University of Pittsburgh School of Nursing, Pittsburgh, PA

1 Visions of Leadership

Becoming a leader is serious stuff. Yet what is leadership? Let's start by suggesting that leadership begins with leading self. A narrative is helpful to set the scene. Rebecca is a health visitor working with a young mother.

She writes: I first meet Tanya when her baby is eleven days old. Discharged from the care of the community midwife on day ten, this is her first health visitor contact. For many women at this stage, this must seem like yet another new health professional to get to know and trust. Before I had had a chance to ring the bell, the front door is opened quickly by a woman who introduced herself as Tanya's mother. I am ushered into the sitting room with a sense of urgency and then left alone with Tanya. She sits on the sofa surrounded by the paraphernalia of parenthood – muslins, creams, napples, bottles, pads and wipes. It seems the whole room is taken up by the trappings of a tiny baby. Tanya looks lost and panic stricken in the midst of it all as if she's been cast adrift on an ocean. I sit beside her and simply ask her to tell me how she's feeling. Her story tumbles out, and for the next part of that grey, damp afternoon, I listen to an unfolding story of false hopes and broken dreams, expectations that now lie shattered and dissolved in a sea of tears. The planned minimal-intervention water birth that became an emergency caesarean section. The anticipated natural, intense pleasures of breastfeeds that became painful, frustrating and anxious hours, fuelled by the fear of her infant's poor weight gain. As the rain falls relentlessly against the shiny patio doors, I abandon all planned paperwork and simply listen to the sad tale of a woman who has always had her life so well planned, so controlled, yet now feels so helpless, so lost. I give her very little advice, mindful that once I would have focused on putting things right, on a successful outcome. I am aware of documentation policy and need for standards

(Continued)

but overridden by the needs of Tanya. I have no fear of sanction as I might have had previously.

I am content to allow Tanya to explore her feelings with me, recognising her need to go through this process, even if there can be no happy ending. I suggest that writing down her thoughts and feelings might help her to make some sense of them. She seems surprised at being 'allowed' to set agenda; she expected to be 'told' what to do. On the way back to the surgery, I smile as I am struck by the parallels of my suggestion to Tanya and my own experience of journaling as a way of exploring contradictions between the desirable and what is actual lived experience. I am conscious of being much more available to Tanya than I have been on similar visits in the past. Why is that? Using the 'influences grid' (Johns 2013) helps me to clarify what factors influenced my actions with Tanya.[1] Using the grid creates a space to review myself and reinforce my values. Now, on reflection, I can see that I was mindfully engaged with Tanya, available within the moment, not distant. Using the word 'engaged' is profound. I remember reading work by Davies (1995), who had used the same terminology. I look up her work again and see how well it fits with my own practice vision. She argues that nursing is devalued by being seen as feminine (and medicine given dominance by its masculinity); although society values nurses, it devalues the caring act of nursing. Can that still be true? I suspect it is. She suggests a gender-free definition of nursing, with characteristics that are a fusion of both masculine and feminine qualities in a non-gendered profession:

- Neither distant nor involved but engaged
- Neither autonomous nor passive/dependent but interdependent
- Neither self-orientated nor self-effacing but accepting of an embodied use of self as part of the therapeutic encounter
- Neither instrumental nor passive but a creator of an active community in which solutions can be negotiated
- Neither master/possessor of knowledge nor the user of experience but a reflective user of experience and expertise

Davies helps me visualise my role as a leader. It offers substance in that I know better what it is I am trying to do leading myself within my practice.

So how does this brief narrative reflect my leadership? Most significantly, it is about relationship. I shift from being authoritative to

(Continued)

facilitative.[2] I resonate with the idea of creating an 'active community' with Tanya and with my other mothers and with my colleagues. Neither did I become so involved with Tanya that the issue became mine, nor so distant that I seemed uncaring, but balanced these two extremes with an active engagement. Pinar (1981: 178) cautions that empathy 'conceals as it reveals', potentially creating a political eunuch if over-involvement results in complicity with another's delusions. Understanding my actions from this deeper, more critical level, embracing organisational and cultural perspectives alongside the aesthetic, helps me deconstruct the experience and recognise ways to sustain it. I could not help but draw comparisons between my responses here, with Cassie in the 'Troubled Minds' narrative I wrote some months earlier. When I was not able to 'fix' Cassie, control her feelings, I could see no role for myself and quickly withdrew. Here, with Tanya, I was able to stay in the moment, available to Tanya without my own agenda, consciously aware of us together, managing the unfolding moment and supporting her in her crisis. This is true presence – bringing humanness to the moment while simultaneously giving self to the other who is exploring the meaning of the situation (Liehr 1989).

Becoming a leader has been more of an unconscious act – others have seen and noted changes, but I have not been so aware of them myself. It is like a child growing –others see her grow, but the child does not notice. The changes occur daily, imperceptibly tiny, barely there, yet cumulative. Being with Tanya I actually felt myself grow, was actively mindful of the process and could feel the transformation. The reflexive spiral is sometimes a gradual unfolding experience and sometimes a dramatic moment of revelation (Johns 2013) – this was my dramatic moment.

Vision

Rebecca's story gives insight into her leadership journey at a particular moment. Mindful of her leadership vision she seeks to live it as a reality. This tension between her vision and her reality is the focus of reflection. Theory opens a dialogical space for Rebecca to reflect on in the context of her experience and informs her practice. Through reflection she can assimilate theory into practice.[3] In this sense, theory adds substance to any leadership vision quest.

3

Vision gives purpose and motivation to action. Whilst every leader should be very clear about their personal vision, such a vision should not be prescribed or imposed. Working in organisations, the idea that a leadership vision should be truly your own might be problematic if no one else agrees with it. Multiple visions at variance with each other by different team members might see everyone pulling in different directions. Imagine being led under such circumstance. I suspect many readers will know this scenario and its morale-deflating consequence.

In constructing a vision of leadership, leaders like Rebecca are cognizant of ideas about leadership. One approach is simply to adopt one idea, for example Bass's ideas of transformational leadership. This approach is compelling because such ideas are comprehensive and authoritative. A more constructive approach is to construct an eclectic vision developed from different sources. This approach requires more thinking and perhaps lacks authority. Yet always the leader must ask, 'What do these theory words mean as something lived?' Only then can the leader move through ideas into a vision of leadership that is truly her own. And even then, the vision is a moveable feast because it is always shifting in light of reflection on its nature. Reviewing the contemporary health care literature on leadership, the idea of transformational leadership is widely viewed as desirable for health care in stark contrast with the prevailing transactional-type leadership characteristic of health care organisations (Bass 1990, Sofarelli and Brown 1998). Sofarelli and Brown (1998) consider that transformational leadership is the model that will assist nursing to develop into an empowered profession with the potential to be a dominant voice in reshaping the health care system of the future.

However, other ideas of leadership need consideration, notably servant leadership. Servant leadership offers a radically different perspective whereby the leader is servant-first in contrast with leader-first. The role of leadership is to literally service those who deliver the service. Imagine how that type of leadership would shift the nature of relationships within the organisation. Playing with ideas is creative, itself a quality of leadership.

Wheatley writes (1999: 130):

> Behaviours don't change by announcing new values. We move only gradually into being able to act congruently with those values. To do this we have to develop much greater awareness of how we're acting; we have to become far more self-reflective than normal ... little by little, tested by events and crises, we learn how to enact these new values. We develop different patterns of behaviour. We slowly become who we said we wanted to be.

'Far more self-reflective than normal' leads into being mindful.

Mindfulness

Kabat-Zin (1994: 76) writes:

> You will need a vision that is truly your own – one that is deep and tenacious and that lies close to the core of who you believe yourself to be, what you value in your life, and where you see yourself going. Only the strength of such a dynamic vision and the motivation from which it springs can possibly keep you on this path year in and year out, with a willingness to practice every day and to bring mindfulness to bear on whatever is happening, to open to whatever is perceived, and to let it point to where the holding is and where the letting go and the growing need to happen.

Kabat-Zin's emphasis on mindfulness is key. Goldstein (2002: 32) describes mindfulness as 'the quality of paying full attention to the moment, opening to the truth of change'. It is the ability to see ourselves clearly without distortion, without judgement. Most of the time our heads are full of 'stuff'. Our minds are everywhere, we get distracted. We don't see things clearly. Leaders learn to empty their minds. As Susuki (1999: 21) writes, 'If your mind is empty, it is always ready for anything; it is open to everything. In the beginner's mind there are many possibilities; in the expert's mind there are few.'

Mindfulness involves the capacity to hold the creative tension between a vision of leadership and realising the vision as a lived reality. It is one thing to have an idea of something and quite another to know it as something truly lived. Being mindful is a reflexive self-awareness, a constant and natural self-inquiry and action towards realising one's leadership values (or vision) as a lived reality. The mindful leader is aware of her assumptions and the way these assumptions influence her perceptions. It is like looking at self in a mirror, warts and all! People undoubtedly smudge the mirror to distort their reflected images to fit in with an ideal self. To see self clearly the mindful leader continuously cleans the mirror even though the images may be uncomfortable. The illusions we hold about ourselves are torn away to reveal the naked self. We wear masks for reasons of sustaining our self-identity. If our masks are pulled away how do we protect our vulnerability? This is the work of reflection, the art of paying attention to self in order to see one's reality and shift this as necessary to become a true leader. However, accessing, critiquing and shifting one's assumptions are not easy because they are socially constructed and experienced as normal through patterns of relationships. If I were to shift my assumptions it would impact on others, creating disturbance in the normal flow of everyday practice.

Every experience is unique, a mystery unfolding. It has not been experienced before although the leader may recognise similar experiences.

Once we think we know we only see what we know. The mind closes to possibility.

Whilst being mindful is the quality of paying attention to what is unfolding NOW, it is, however, attached to a sense of both the future and the past. With regard to the future, leadership is purposeful; the leader constantly holds the intent to realise her vision of leadership. With regard to the past, I find the Buddhist word *apramada* helpful. It means the guardian at the gate of the senses ever alert to threat. Sangharakshita (1988: 148) writes, 'all the time, inattention and errors are trying to get hold of us, but our mind, keeping alert all the time, is trying to drive them away'. So whilst the mind is purposeful it is also clearing away obstacles to achieving that purpose. Greenleaf (2002: 41) alludes to mindfulness as a quality of leadership – 'The cultivation of awareness gives one the basis for detachment, the ability to stand aside and see oneself in perspective in the context of one's own experience, amid the ever present dangers, threats and alarms.' It is through reflection that the leader becomes increasingly aware of self within her practice, more aware of the way she thinks, feels and responds, more aware of her purpose and more aware of those forces that constrain her achievement. In this way, mindfulness is nurtured.

Transforming and transformational leadership

The founding father of transformational leadership is James McGregor Burns. He coined the idea of a transforming leadership necessary for a just and increasingly complex global society, moving the idea of leadership away from previous theories of leadership based on trait, behaviour or tasks (Northouse 2001) and situational theory (Hersey and Blanchard 1982).

Burns (1978: 20) writes, 'Transforming leadership occurs when one person engages with others in such a way that the leader and follower raise one another to higher levels of motivation and morality.' This brief description is inspirational in its clarity and brevity. It opens a path to sensing leadership as something lived as relational, moral and mutually empowering. Every action the leader takes is purposeful towards creating a better world.

Emerging from the foundational work of Burns, Bass (1985) developed transformational leadership that was related more to organisational leadership than to Burns' wider social agenda. Bass set out four interrelated essential aspects of transformational leadership that offer a dynamic framework to appreciate its fundamental nature:

- Idealised influence – that leadership is based on genuine trust built on a moral foundation.

- Inspirational motivation – that leadership provides meaning and challenge for engaging others in working collaboratively towards shared goals and success.
- Intellectual stimulation – that leadership liberates the creative and responsive spirit in followers to fulfil their individual and collective aspirations towards overcoming problems in realising a shared vision.
- Individual consideration – that leadership invests in each person towards enabling the person to fulfil their potential and needs leading to higher achievement and growth.

These four aspects are concerned with the relationship between the leader and her followers. Words like 'genuine trust', 'engaging', 'moral foundation', 'meaning', 'collaboration', 'shared goals', 'success', 'creativity', 'aspirations', 'shared vision', 'invests', 'higher achievement' and 'growth' are powerful. A transformational leadership culture brings out the best in people – people are happier, more satisfied and more responsible. It synergises energy towards greater performance.

This positions leadership as essentially an ontological concern, in contrast with an epistemological concern with ideas and tasks. The rhetoric of empowerment and dominant voice sounds like a holy grail. However, the emphasis on empowerment is pertinent because the ability of nurses, midwives and health visitors to realise leadership may be constrained by a legacy of subordination. A vexing challenge! There have been many interpretations of transformational leadership. In her narrative, Martha utilises Schuster's approach (see Chapter 2).

Bass contrasted transformational leadership with a transactional type of leadership based on contingent reward in exchange for good performance. Performance is managed in one of three essential ways:

- By exception (active) – Watches and searches for deviations from rules and standards and takes corrective action.
- By exception (passive) – Intervenes only if standards are not met.
- Laissez-faire – Abdicates responsibilities and avoids making decisions.

The transactional nature lies in the exchange – reward in exchange for effort. The supervisory nature of active management by exception reflects the command and control behaviour where the focus is on outcome rather than process. The passive mode reflects a managerial indifference unless outcomes are blatantly not being met, usually noted at times of audit or complaint. It leads to a mediocrity of performance. Both active and passive forms of management are not conducive to good relationships. Such management patterns are essentially mindless and lived on

7

autopilot, operating on assumptions that have not been challenged for a long time (Gilley 1997).

The transformational and transactional are essentially different ways of being in the world. They are not different hats to wear at different times. Otherwise transformational leadership would be instrumental and inauthentic. Transactional leadership is not a fall-back position for when transformational leadership falters. I must be clear. In my view there is no such thing as transactional leadership. Perhaps 'commander' or 'controller' would be a more suitable word than 'leader' in the transactional world. Command and control are the antithesis of leadership, concerned as it is with producing specific outcomes in contrast with leadership's quest to enable growth through human relationships.

The transactional pyramid

The transactional organisation is symbolised as a pyramid layered through a rigid set of hierarchical- and bureaucratic-bound levels (Figure 1.1). The pyramid symbolises a top-down approach structured through managerial roles governed by rules of engagement, status and positional power. At its apex, the transactional organisation has a mission statement written as a set of strategic objectives set largely by political demand and wrapped in ideological rhetoric. The vision is interpreted as targets or outcomes. The organisation is either rewarded or punished by its success in meeting these strategic objectives at all costs. Because of this demand, the whole

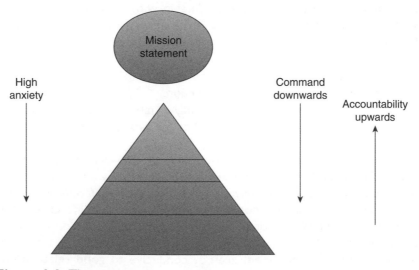

Figure 1.1 The transactional pyramid

pyramid is infused with high anxiety transmitted downward through its hierarchical levels. When people are anxious they must try to control their environment in an effort to manage anxiety resulting in command and control behaviour. It demands team players yet sets the rules for team play that constantly change in response to organisational anxiety, often without consultation with those affected by such rules. As often heard, 'the goal posts are always changing'. Little emphasis is given to how these targets or outcomes will be met in terms of process. Inevitably, a strong emphasis on outcomes reduces people to 'resources' to meet targets. It is a dehumanising system that evokes low morale, distrust and compliance to avoid sanction. The whole pyramid functions on elaborate systems that demand adherence. When things go wrong it is blamed on human error rather than the system. The system can be viewed as a complex machine – a Newtonian mechanistic perspective of the world with an emphasis on its own smooth running (Freidson 1970). The transactional organisation does not like assertive people because they may disturb the status quo, sending ripples across its smooth running. Power within transactional organisations such as the NHS has a typical authoritative pattern to ensure a *docile and competent workforce* (Foucault 1979) – 'docile to the extent that its subordinates do not disrupt its smooth running (Johns 2009: 131)'. Perhaps most of all, its managers believe they are effective leaders. Yet when organisational managers are observed, the delusion of leadership is easily revealed, especially around taking risks and giving away power.[4] Delusion is an immense boulder to shift. It is like asking a nurse if she is caring. To say 'no' would be shocking. Locked into its tightly bound systems the transactional organisation cannot let go and unfold into a transformational culture simply because it would destroy itself. This is all about survival. Crippled by its anxiety, the transactional organisation disempowers its staff through its patterns of relationship. People are pawns in a game to be moved around the board at the mercy of the chess master in his or her omnipotence. It projects its anxiety into people, criticising and blaming unreasonably behind an internalised sense of threat that serves to keep people in their place. It is a culture of fear and oppression. It does not realise its impact on others, or if it does, it doesn't see it as a problem.

Leadership is not management

Let's get one thing clear – leadership is *not* management. Management is essentially *doing* certain sorts of tasks whereas leadership is *being* a certain sort of person. The shift from doing to being lifts leadership into the human encounter. It is not about *what I do*, as *I am* is some sort of object, but *who I am* in relationship with others. For this reason, leadership does not lend

9

itself to a reduction into competencies although the quest to know leadership often results in such outcome.

In a world where leadership does not exist it is easy to imagine that management is leadership. Then when you see another view, the realisation drops like a lead weight. Management is getting the job done to an agreed quality in line with targets and resources, including ensuring and managing the necessary resources. It is a business arrangement, a transaction between the organisation and its workers. I wonder, must leaders who are managers necessarily wear two hats? I think not. It does not require different personas. Yet, in positioning themselves within their organisations, the leaders must appreciate the tension between any idealised notion of leadership and the reality of their managerial role.

Luke is a senior nurse working in an accident and emergency department.

He writes: I realise that my initial impression of what constituted leadership was not leadership at all, but rather management. I viewed leadership as someone in a position of power with strong opinions who demanded respect. Examination of the literature on leadership revealed a more appealing, inspirational view of leadership. It is hoped by differentiating leadership from management, the basis for understanding true leadership begins – 'managers are people who often work in hierarchical organisations and are in positions which have legitimate sources of power with the authority to delegate. The emphasis of their work lies in control, decision making, decision analysis and results' (Marquis and Huston 1996). Within a hierarchical organisation like the NHS, the manager described above is instantly recognisable where the emphasis is on authority, power, control and decision making.

The transformational organisation

In contrast to the pyramidal transactional organisation, a transformational organisation is represented as a round table where colleagues come together to co-create meaningful work based on a shared vision towards shared success (Figure 1.2).

Each person around the table, no matter their role, is viewed as an equal, respected and valued for their particular role within the whole. Although there is a designated leader, the leader is intent on each person who sits at the table becoming a leader in their own right, whereby each person assumes responsibility for his or her own performance towards realising the shared

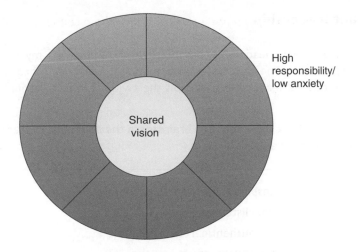

High
responsibility/
low anxiety

Shared
vision

Figure 1.2 The transformational leadership round table

vision and for ensuring the whole group works collaboratively. It might be expected that an emphasis on responsibility could create increased anxiety. This is mitigated by the impact of team support to create a low-anxiety learning environment that views conflict or difference in views as a learning opportunity in contrast with the transactional blame-and-shame culture. It is the idea of every person taking responsibility that is profoundly difficult when emerging from a transactional climate of subordination. Taking responsibility for self and the group is demanding. It is standing up and being counted. It is a demand for commitment to working collaboratively with others.

Becoming a leader is not a rational process of shifting one's mindset from a transactional to a transformational perspective. This shift is a culture shock because health care organisations must inevitably resist a trans-formational-type leadership because it does not fit smoothly within its transactional culture. This creates a tension between a vision of leadership and realising the vision as a lived reality. Understanding and resolving this *creative* tension is the learning focus for becoming a leader. No easy task for an individual leader given the weight of the organisation. As such, realising leadership is not so much an individual thing, but something that needs to be nurtured within an organisational culture that values and lives leadership as a way of organisational relationship. From this perspective, leadership must be consistently role modelled, establishing a leadership culture that nurtures others to become leaders. As Covey warns (2002: 2), 'We've got to produce more for less and with greater speed than we've ever done before. The only way to do that is through the empowerment of people.'

Servant leadership

Discovering servant leadership has profoundly influenced my vision of leadership, moving me beyond transformational leadership into a more practical model of leadership based on the twin ideas of community and service.

In one exercise I ask the leaders to brainstorm the attributes of leadership. Many words are generated:

> inspiring, motivating, charismatic
>
> mindful, listens well, just, fair, challenging
>
> authentic, real, vulnerable
>
> mutual respect, collaborative
>
> confident yet not arrogant
>
> available, approachable
>
> intentional, trusting, responsible
>
> invests in people, empowering
>
> caring, visionary, compassionate, humble
>
> realistic and focused, credible, walks the talk
>
> getting results that matter (realising organisational objectives)
>
> moral (towards creating better worlds)
>
> powerful, charismatic
>
> patience, wisdom, expert
>
> human!
>
> spiritual
>
> community
>
> service

I add *community* and *service* to the list. The significance of each of the qualities is explored. I ask, 'Do you have these attributes?' 'Do people you work with have these attributes?' Perhaps, for the first time, the aspiring leaders look into the mirror of self.

The idea of community and service as defining qualities of leadership in a dominant transactional culture is both radical and utter sense. The idea of service is that the leader leads from behind turning upside down the conventional idea that leaders lead from the front. If taken seriously, it fundamentally shifts the power relationship within the organisation. As Gilley (1997: 41) writes, 'When leaders take a second, closer look, they see that the lines between groups of people blur. The leaders begin to see that although their employers serve them, they must also serve the employees.'

Where to draw the line? For myself, as leader of a community hospital, the line was drawn by the decision to utilise primary nursing as the mode of care delivery whereby the individual primary nurse takes responsibility for her patients. My role as leader was both to support the nurses to take responsibility for their performance and to enable them to develop that performance. To do so, I had to let go of control (power).

Greenleaf (2002: 13–14) writes:

> The servant leader is servant first. It begins with the natural feeling that one wants to serve, to serve first. Then conscious choice brings one to aspire to lead. That person is sharply different from one who is leader first, perhaps because of the need to assuage an unusual power drive or to acquire material possessions. The leader-first and the servant-first are two extreme types. Between them there are shadings and blends that are part of the infinite variety of human nature. The difference manifests itself in the care taken by the servant-first to make sure that other people's highest priority needs are being served. The best test, and difficult to administer, is: Do those served grow as persons? Do they, while being served, become healthier, wiser, freer, more autonomous, more likely themselves to become servants?

The defining nature of servant leadership is servant-first in contrast with leader-first. Whilst servant leadership has much in common with a transformational leadership, it is radical because it turns the transactional pyramid upside down and shakes out all its power symbols.

The leader-first usually sits at the head of the table whilst the servant-first might sit at the foot of the table, ensuring that all at the table are well served. Both might espouse collaborative intent but would approach it very differently. Servant leadership acknowledges that the most important people are those who deliver care – this is why the organisation exists. It takes leadership into a profound new dimension, one that is not easy to grasp, let alone accommodate within the prevailing transactional landscape.

As a holistic therapist, I can appreciate the idea of being of service as I kneel at the client's feet with the intention of helping and guiding them towards better health. This is energetic work. Leaders are adept at centring their energy to lift others beyond their normal limits towards greatness. Rael draws attention to a universal energy that the leader knows how to tune into and utilise. He writes (1993: 88–9), 'when it [consciousness] begins to lift to a higher level, something dramatic can happen'.

You, the reader, will know this: the way some people lift you and others drain you. It is as if people radiate energy, some infusing, some depleting. Patients also know this: those nurses who lift them and those who do not. I wonder how much better patients would heal if all nurses radiated this lifting energy? How much money would be saved? How much better nurses themselves would feel. Leaders know and nurture this energy. They are the great 'lifters'. They invest in themselves so they can lift as a natural aspect of their being. It is not a tap to turn on as if an offensive charm. Leaders know how to centre their energy and grow from their exchanges with followers. As I sit around the 'team table' I am mindful of 'who I am', offering my view, challenging and inspiring others, opening the imagination, moving people towards realising our collective vision of hospice. I visualise myself as a peacemaker. As Jones and Jones write (1996: 135), 'From a sea full of problems, leaders [peacemakers] find solutions. They honour the trail ahead and know that a path of least resistance exists. They focus on the possible.'

I sense that servant leadership has much in common with Buddhism – essentially, a wise and compassionate response to the other's suffering in ways that enable the person to grow. It is like a vibration that spreads to embrace the whole organisation, a ripple from around the shared collaborative table. Deep within the idea of service is a sense of humility, in the giving of service asking for nothing in reward. This is not a false humility. Of course, serving is its own reward, in seeing both the other and self grow. With humility there is no pretence. The leader is honest and vulnerable – not anxious that he might be exposed as a fraud. Servant leadership resonates with what Prosser (2010) refers to as post-heroic leadership, reflected in such work as *Authentic leadership* (George 2003), *Leading quietly* (Badaracco 2002) and the qualities of the level 5 leader portrayed in *Good to great* – such qualities as being modest, inspiring, selfless and praiseworthy (Collins 2001).

In his book *Servant leadership* Greenleaf sets out the qualities of the servant leader. This work reflects Greenleaf's anecdotal stance rather than claiming validity for his approach through any research. Perhaps the whole idea of service has a romantic feel in stark contrast with the dominant transactional health care culture. As I say to aspiring leaders, it may be a step too far just now, yet be inspired by it, and yet more and more of the aspiring leaders choose this vision of leadership to guide them. Why? Because it is essentially a mindful approach.

Community

Leaders do not work alone. They create communities based on mutual support and respect, trust, commitment, responsibility and love. The circle best symbolises community rather like King Arthur's legendary round table or the Native American powwow. Ideally people sit wherever around the table to avoid symbolising one particular place as the power chair. Community is the basis of the collaborative team that works together to realise its collective vision. It is a place of belonging and growth.

Initiative

Leaders take the initiative! They 'take the risk of failure along with the chance of success'. (Greenleaf 2002: 29). They hold the vision and a sustaining spirit to support the movement towards realising the vision. They are good at pointing the direction. Greenleaf (2002: 29) writes,

> They [leaders] are better than most at pointing the direction. As long as one is leading, one always has a goal. It may be a goal arrived at by group consensus, or the leader, acting on inspiration, may simply have said, 'Let's go this way'. But the leader always knows what it is and can articulate it for those who are unsure. By clearly stating the goal the leader gives certainty to others who may have difficulty in achieving it for themselves.

Leaders listen. Greenleaf asks, 'Why is there so little listening?' Through listening, the leader comes to truly appreciate the situation and can respond rather than react. Listening is one thing, speaking is another. Just being there for others and listening to them is one of the most important capacities a leader can have (Jaworski 1998: 67). The leader is a master of language and imagination. It is the facility 'in tempting the hearer into that leap of imagination that connects the verbal concept to the hearer's own experience' (Greenleaf 2002: 32). Withdrawal is about the leader taking time out to charge energy to keep self at an optimum level of performance. To serve others one has to be in good shape. Service is not sacrifice! Acceptance and empathy indicate that the leader is always open to receive. Acceptance is a tolerance to imperfection, although not an acceptance of lack of responsibility. Empathy reflects the facility and willingness to connect with people's experience. Only then can the leader understand. Leaders are focused on who they are and what they need to do. They do not get sidetracked into peripheral issues and waste energy on futile actions. Leaders organise life simply because they have the facility to raise the spirit of the people around a clear articulation of necessary action.

The leader throws open the doors of awareness and perception, drawing on all her senses to get the big picture. As Greenleaf writes (2002: 33), 'The cultivation of awareness gives one the basis for detachment, the ability to stand aside and see oneself in perspective in the context of ones own experience.' This idea of awareness and empathy towards self resonates with being mindful, the hallmark of leadership.

Foresight

Foresight gives leaders their leading edge. Greenleaf (2002: 21–22) writes, '[The leader] needs to have a sense for the unknowable and be able to foresee the unforeseeable. Leaders know some things and foresee some things which those they are presuming to lead do not know or foresee as clearly. This is partly what gives leaders their lead, what puts them out ahead and qualifies them to show the way.'

Foresight has a somewhat mystical quality. It resonates with the idea of chaos theory (Wheatley 1999) that somehow the leader can tune into the patterning around meaning and intention. It is about processing what is happening now, informed by the past and anticipating the future. I might call this wisdom the ability to weigh up the situation even before it unfolds and know how best to respond considering the consequences.

Foresight is possible when the leader is able to process information towards making best decisions in both the short and long term. It is not being attached to knowing and being open to the possibility of the moment. Foresight is faith in oneself that followers know and trust. Salzberg (2002: 67) writes of faith,

> It doesn't decide how we are going to perceive something but rather is the ability to move forward even without knowing. In order to deepen our faith, we have to be able to carry things out, to wonder, to doubt. In fact, faith is strengthened by doubt when doubt is sincere, critical questioning combined with a deep trust in our own right and ability to discern the truth.

Persuasion

Although leaders often have positional power as befits their position within the organisational hierarchy, they do not emphasise this type of power and certainly avoid coercion. Instead, they give emphasis to expert and relational power, what French and Raven (1968) describe as facilitative power,[5] whilst reinforcing intrinsic reward by appealing to values and responsibility.

Key principles of servant leadership

Considering Greenleaf's characteristics I established eight key princi-ples of servant leadership. I added the dimensions of perseverance and poise, qualities I consider vital to leadership but which Greenleaf does not give overt attention. These eight principles are set out in Chapter 4 as a prelude to Alison's narrative in which she endeavours to realise servant leadership.

Against this theoretical background I will now explore broader, more philo-sophic ideas of leadership: leadership as chaos, leadership as feminine and leadership as caring.

Leadership as chaos

Chaos theory challenges the idea of an orderly and predicable world upon which the transactional organisation is predicated, reflected in its demand for smooth running as its *sine qua non*. This suggests a Newtonian machine – like mentality. A machine comprises many parts and, as with any machine when it doesn't function well, the emphasis is on fixing the part or parts that are problematic. Within this machine metaphor, people become part of the machine and are naturally blamed for any malfunction – what might be called the human factor. Management's primary role is to ensure the smooth running.

In contrast, chaos theory views the world as a whole, mindful of the rela-tionship between parts. Only by seeing the whole can things be understood. This is the leader's perspective. Chaos theory accepts the world is funda-mentally chaotic and not easily predicted within the complexity and uncer-tainty of everyday human experience. Targets can only ever be speculative and misleading because they have traditionally focused action. Yet every-thing is always changing. There is an inherent order within chaos framed around the idea of meaning, what are known as strange attractors (Wheat-ley 1999). From this perspective, the leader can relax control, knowing that things will work out just fine based on practice values. Practice becomes self-organising. There is a creative edge between stability and instability that is important for the leader to read and tread. On this edge everything is in flux, dynamic and changeable. The transactional world, fearful of conse-quences, clings to stability, leading to a static and sterile work environment. There is a natural synergy between mindfulness and chaos theory – that to tread the creative edge of chaos the leader must be mindful. It won't work otherwise. Indeed it will be a disaster.

17

Leadership as feminine

Leadership might be viewed as a feminine approach to organisation in con-trast with a more masculine approach that characterises the transactional organisation. The work of Gilligan (1982), *In a Different Voice*, gives sub-stance to this gender contrast. In her research she noted that men and women have different ethical values. From Gilligan's perspective a feminine leadership is grounded in responsibility and relationships whereas a mas-culine-type leadership is grounded in justice based on rationality and rules.

Heather was attracted to a transformational leadership because she sensed it resonated with her feminine caring values. She sought congruence between her leadership and being a woman.

> She writes: Rosener (1990) writes that women tend to prefer transformational approaches to leadership. Wedderburn-Tate (1999) writes, however, that the current environment of our health care system – finance-driven, performance attainment, short-term initiatives and territorial battles – is not conducive to producing transformative leaders. This seems to suggest that women who desire to be leaders often suffer a sense of conflict between personal and professional expectations. Are female leaders socialised then into behaving in a certain way to 'fit in'? Barker and Young (1994) write of the continuing domination of patriarchal values and assumptions where competition, control and manipulation are the predominant (transactional) influ-ences in the modern world. They suggest that as the post-modern period develops, there will be an increasing emphasis on feminine values and beliefs, such as caring, nurturing and intuition, to balance patriarchal views. The modern and post-modern world are today oper-ating side by side and in conflict at present. The transition in thinking is slowly happening but is not predicted to be complete for another 10–20 years (Barker and Young 1994). Challenges and tension seemed to lie ahead if I aimed to be true to myself and learn the skills necessarily to provide the desirable practice of transformational leadership that fits comfortably with my own feminist caring ethics of nursing within this harsh, primarily transactional, environment.

Barker and Young's prediction was written twenty years ago. Since that time I sense no discernible movement towards a more feminine leadership. Perhaps you, the reader, will discern it differently? Perhaps there are more women in senior management, but does that equate with feminine values? Patriarchal

Right brain Masculine Yang		Left brain Feminine Yin
Reason Rationality Justice Order Logic	B A L A N C E	Perception Imagination Creativity Intuition Empathy Wonder

Table 1.1 Contrasting right and left brain qualities

structures are immensely thick, hewn over the years and supported by a government bent on a target approach to health care despite the numerous health warnings of failed care. As such, framing leadership as feminine may not serve the cause of leadership within the dominant patriarchal organisational culture. As Rebecca explored, Davies (1995) argues that nursing is devalued by being seen as feminine (and medicine given dominance by its masculinity); although society values nurses, it devalues the caring act of nursing.

The feminine is often associated with the right side of the brain, the masculine with the left side of the brain (Table 1.1) – Yin and Yang. The transactional world reflects the masculine with an emphasis on rationality, reason, justice and order, whilst the feminine reflects an emphasis on perception, imagination, intuition, creativity, empathy and wonder – all qualities vital for leadership that are nurtured through leadership coaching using humanities and art. It is significant to acknowledge that the transformational is not opposite to the transactional but accommodates it in seeking wholeness.

The leader uses the whole brain and achieves greatness (Woolf 1945). In other words, the leader finds synergy between her masculine and feminine side. Both masculine and feminine qualities are significant for effective leadership. It is interesting to speculate whether one side should mediate the other. Hence men as leaders would naturally lean to the right and women naturally lean to the left. Being mindful, the leader appreciates this interplay. This phenomenon is most visible in men who have undertaken the leadership programme perhaps because women are naturally socialised to embrace the masculine given its domination.

Marge writes: Choosing to become a leader led me to embark upon a voyage of self-examination and self-discovery, arousing feelings of restlessness and impatience, which has driven me to question my previous acceptance and acquiescence in the role of wife and mother. My dual identity as a woman and professional nurse presents me with a personal dilemma, because as a senior nurse and a woman, I find myself working in a male-oriented professional health care system where masculine values, particularly those of doctors and senior managers, appear to be viewed as more significant and dominant and thus attain priority in the primary care trust (PCT) in which I am employed. These attitudes and values are becoming increasingly incompatible with my family life and responsibilities. When I am at work, in my professional persona, I now find myself considering whether as a senior nurse I aspire to have masculine values within the PCT. This causes immense contradiction, in recognition that in doing so, I face continual denial of self and alienation from my nursing colleagues, and yet behaving as the ideal woman and nurse and perpetuating expected perceived norms, I risk experiencing the suppression of voice in my personal and professional life and this leaves me feeling incredibly uncomfortable. This exploration of discomfort and frustration forms the basis of my journey. In recognition that I must be courageous and reveal to my reader who I think I am, at my starting point, I capture the flavours of the text from an early entry from within my reflective journal. I begin with this fearful attempt of looking inwards, to a place of freedom from distraction, as I contemplate self in the turmoil of my work as a senior nurse and as a mother and wife to my family. In my current senior nurse position, where I have been for the past five months, only now that I am standing back can I appreciate how much I enjoyed my previous position in contrast to where I now find self. I question whether where I am is in tune with my values and beliefs, as I am uncertain about my commitment to this role as nurse manager, if it means that I am to be like my colleagues: desiring to be at the centre of the action as 'the captain' and expected to work incredibly long hours, to be part of the internal race and to be seen to be the first in the office and the last to leave! Can I cope with only being allowed to be covertly compassionate, ensuring that compassion is not obviously displayed by self as a manager, as it seems that by 'showing I care' is a weakness I bring with me? Does caring for others and valuing people stop me from earning the right as a senior to credibly 'run the show'?

(Continued)

And so I question whether my self-esteem has been flattened by coming here, at a time when in the context of my new status I should be respected for who I am and the personal and professional qualities I bring, not my ability to conform with the values of colleagues. I find myself faced with two choices. I can either collaborate with their established ways of relating and be like them or maintain a conscious awareness and sensitivity of dynamics within the organisation, by being mindful and less harsh on self, so that I can behave in tune with my values and beliefs and in doing so begin to redefine my position as a manger within this organisation and live a congruent life, not a façade.

Sharing these words within her leadership community evoked strong feelings and opinions for it seemed to get to the very heart of becoming a leader and the tensions women, in particular, confronted, when they were prepared to face it. It seems that to succeed in a patriarchal culture one must embrace patriarchal values, especially if you are a woman – as if to prove you are serious about management. Not to do so, to turn against the grain, puts you out of kilter and makes you ultimately not management material.

Women's way of knowing

The feminist perspective can be expanded by appreciating the work of Belenky et al. (1986), who established a typology of different levels of knowing. They framed women's empowerment through five levels from which women view reality: silence, received voice, subjective voice, procedural voice and constructed knowing (Table 1.2).

Constructed voice	
Procedural voice – separate and connected voices	
Subjective voice	Empowerment ↑
Received voice	
Silence	

Table 1.2 Women's ways of knowing self through voice

Silence – reflecting how many women in transactional organisations are socialised to be silenced by patriarchal oppression. It is a position of subjugation and powerlessness that constrains the emergence of self-identity. The Cumberlege Report (Department of Health and Social Security, 1986), which reviewed the future of community health care, noted that in meetings doctors filled the front rows and asked all the questions whilst nurses filled the back rows and were silent. Cumberlege noted that if nursing was ever to emerge as a profession it needed to find its voice. How many meetings do you attend where people are silent? What reasons govern such silence?

The received voice – where women speak with a given voice – reflecting that they have no voice of their own. They speak what is expected of them and are not required to think or speak for themselves. How often do people say, 'Tell me what I need to know?' How often do health care practitioners endeavour to solve problems for people by telling them what they need to do? The received voice reflects a dominant transmission of knowledge – informing people what they need to know, where knowledge and language constitute power.

The subjective voice – what Belenky et al. (1986: 76) describe as the 'quest for self'. At this level women express views and opinions that are largely unsubstantiated and hence easily dismissed. This voice is vital and is the voice most expressed as the aspiring leaders commence their leadership journey. It is the voice nurtured within the leadership community.

The procedural voice has two aspects – the separate and connected voices that mirror the right–left brain dichotomy. Returning to the idea of the masculine and feminine, the separate voice is masculine and the connected voice feminine. The patient is reduced to an object subjected to theory rather than remaining a sentient human being. Leadership likewise can be reduced to the application of science and people objects towards meeting predicted outcomes. Both voices are vital for leadership and yet so much emphasis is given within educational organisations to valuing and developing the separate voice. As a consequence people tend to be lopsided and lean to the left side. The two sides of procedural knowing may antagonise each other – the separate knower may disdain the connected self in the belief 'so that flowers of pure reason may flourish' Belenky et al. (1986: 109). In a health care culture dominated by a demand for a science of prediction, the connected voice is easily diminished.

The constructed voice is the synthesis of the separate and connected voices (Table 1.3). This voice is informed, caring and assertive although not necessarily heard along the transactional corridors. Hence it must be political and persistent. The constructed voice is the voice of leadership. Being assertive is to know the political game and fearlessly push the boundaries yet without

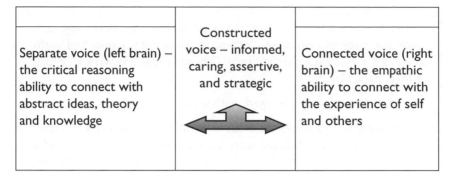

Separate voice (left brain) – the critical reasoning ability to connect with abstract ideas, theory and knowledge	Constructed voice – informed, caring, assertive, and strategic	Connected voice (right brain) – the empathic ability to connect with the experience of self and others

Table 1.3 The synthesis of procedural voices to establish the constructed voice

tripping up and marginalising self as 'difficult'. In pushing the boundaries the leader teaches, encourages and rewards people to develop a constructive voice necessary for effective dialogue.

Leadership as caring

Rebecca drew on the work of Davies to help her visualise her leadership role in being with Tanya. From her reflection, caring emerges as a synthesis of the masculine and feminine; neither one nor the other but a constructed knowing as Belenky et al. (1986).

Perhaps the emphasis on leadership as feminine naturally lends itself to the idea of leadership as caring. Lord Darzi (2008: 11) in the *High quality care for all* report Department of Health 2008: 11 states: 'High quality care should be safe and effective as possible, with compassion, dignity and respect. As well as clinical quality and safety, quality means care that is personal to each individual.'

Lord Darzi gives some meaning to the idea of caring. The word 'compassion' reflects how caring is viewed as a kind of focused love. To be compassion is to have room in your heart for the other's suffering (Levine 1988), not to be confused with sympathy. However, such is the paucity of compassion in health care that a Scottish project entitled 'Leadership in Compassionate Care' was established (Adamson et al. 2009). Perhaps one reason for low morale amongst NHS staff is the inability to be compassionate due to the transactional nature of health care that reduces people to objects, both staff and patients. Is it a failure of leadership if staff lack compassion? I think so.

23

Rachael writes: I have learnt that leadership is love. As the ego falls away the door of love opens. Wrapped up in self my love had withered as if a vine on a parched tree. Gibran (1926: 35) writes, 'Work is love made visible'.

He asks, 'And what is it to work with love?'

He answers, 'It is to weave the cloth with the threads drawn from your heart, even as if your beloved were to wear that cloth. It is to build a house with affection even if your beloved were to dwell in that house. It is to sow seeds with tenderness and reap the harvest with joy, even as if your beloved were to eat the fruit.' I recognise the depth of these words, the love, care and nurture required and commitment needed to sustain my passion and create an environment that empowers others to sustain their own passion. If I can work with love, then this will continue to facilitate the learning environment.

Rachael's words are profound although I am sure many readers shy away from the idea of love, yet embrace the idea of compassion. Indeed health care workers are exhorted to be compassionate as if this is some kind of applied skill rather than something heartfelt.[6]

Mayeroff (1971: 1) considers that 'To care for another person, in the most significant sense, is to help him grow and actualise himself.' These words fit well with both transformational and servant leadership – that the key role of leadership is to enable the other person, whether patient or staff member, to grow.

Caring is the attractor working within health care and this must exist at every level of its functioning. If this is true, then working in health care must fundamentally be about caring. When it isn't, the contradiction is stark, and both patients and staff suffer. Whilst I thought that caring should be natural for health care practitioners, the aspiring leaders generally felt that caring, like leadership, was a rare commodity amongst managers and, more worryingly, at the delivery of patient care. This state of affairs is another reflection of poor leadership, with its managerial focus on filling in paper and meeting targets. It is a simple equation: if commanders treat staff as objects towards meeting outcomes, then staff are likely to respond in similar ways to more junior staff and down the line to patients. This is a huge contradiction for organisations whose business is health care.

All health care practitioners, at every level of the organisation, need to be mindful of self as caring. Leaders work within teams towards a collective vision of health care practice within the wider organisation, whose primary concern is health *care*. Leaders create and sustain a creative and moral environment necessary for individual and organisational growth that is *care*. If an organisation expects its people to care it must also care for those people. It is a simple yet profound equation. And yet everywhere I find that people do not feel cared for within their health care organisations. They feel like objects. It leads to a depersonalisation, and the risk is that they then treat patients like objects. Cared-for people become more inspired, motivated, less toxic, work harder, etc. The list of benefits is endless. If people are not cared for, then the opposite can be assumed.

My partner recently had an angiogram. In the course of the morning we met three nurses; neither one introduced herself by name or acknowledged my presence as her partner. Neither did they inquire as to how my partner was feeling, and let's face it, an angiogram and possibility of stent insertion is not something to be taken lightly. In contrast, the consultant introduced himself, acknowledged my presence with a firm handshake and inquired into our feelings. The difference was so stark. We felt cared for by the doctor but had no faith in the nurses. They were like robots. Instead of being cared for, we felt *uncared* for, adding to our suffering (Johns 2014). Why do these nurses respond in this way? The simple answer is lack of leadership. I would like to think that such stories were rare, the exception rather than the rule, but I meet many people who tell similar stories, as if the whole system of health care is infected by its transactional manner. It simply isn't acceptable, especially when the *patient experience* is lauded as a quality measure. Without doubt, leadership is grounded in humanness. As Freire writes (1972: 43), 'It is essential for the oppressed to realise that when they accept the struggle for humanization they also accept, from that moment, their total responsibility for the struggle.'

Mayeroff writes (1971: 2),

> In the context of a man's life, caring has a way of ordering his other values and activities around it. When this ordering is comprehensive, because of the inclusiveness of his caring, there is a basic stability in his life; he is "in place in the world", instead of being "out of place", or merely drifting endlessly seeking his place. Through caring for certain others, by serving them through caring, a man lives his meaning of his own life.

Being a leader is being 'in place in the world' to lead without contradiction. Being in place the person is able to grow. This can be contrasted with being 'out of place' or knowing your place as determined by others within the transactional organisation. It is like being contained within a box slotted into the pyramidal layers. It is restrictive and hinders growth in its demand to conform to rules set by others.

The leadership journey can be viewed as a movement from 'knowing your place' to being 'in place' as a transformational leader. Mayeroff (1971: 9) reveals the delicacy of such movement so as not to fall into the transactional pattern of imposing direction to shape the person to fit the organisation. In helping the other grow I do not impose my own direction; rather, I allow the direction of the other's growth to guide what I do and to help determine how I am to respond.

> Joan writes: 'Knowing your place' is determined by the organisation within the transactional matrix. Being in the right place is determined by the practitioner in terms of creating the practice conditions to realise desirable practice. The leadership plot is to appreciate and shift into the right place. It is a claim for autonomy based on shared success. Yet my struggle is to know my place within the competing organisational demands let alone find my own place! Perhaps that is my predicament – that I am trying like a good girl to know my place, to satisfy my masters, rather than take over the agenda and find the right place to be in.

Front foot thinking

Front foot thinking is about 'being in place', taking the initiative and being proactive, rather than being caught on the back foot, reactive, defensive and uncertain. The leader is mindful of being on the front foot, as if leading the dance, rather than on the back foot being led. In leading the dance, the leader guides followers to dance and become leaders through role modelling.

In Table 1.4 I set out indicators of being on the front or back foot. These have been generated through dialogue with aspiring leaders over time and constantly evolve as we better appreciate the idea. Being proactive resonates with foresight, intuitively knowing what needs to be done at what

Front foot thinking	Back foot thinking
10 9 8 7 6 5 4 3 2 1	
Views self as a leader	Views self as follower
Uses initiative/proactive	Waits for others to command/reactive
Takes responsibility	Shirks responsibility
Assertive/confident	Non-assertive/hesitant

Mindful of being on the 'front foot'	Not aware of being on the 'front foot'
Strong sense of purpose/morality/values	Weak sense of purpose/morality/values
Takes initiative	Lets things slide
Alert/is prepared	Not alert/Unprepared
Visible to others	Keeps head down
Recognises own value	Need others to value them
Focuses on strengths	Focuses on weaknesses
Sees the whole picture	Sees only the picture they want to see
Crosses hierarchical lines	Hierarchy bound
Voice is heard	Voice subdued
Expands autonomy	Shrinks autonomy
Foresight	Hindsight
Thinks outside the box/creative	Thinks inside the box/conforming
Dynamic sense of relationship	Confined by normal relationships
Poised	Anxious
'In the right place'	'Put in place'
Decisive	Prevaricates
Collaborative	Accommodating/avoiding
Bounces back (resilient)	Falls over (fragile)
Engaged	Detached
Yields	Fails
Takes risks/fearless	Plays safe/defensive

Table 1.4 Front foot/back foot thinking

time. It is being a step ahead, the front foot placed with certainty in front. Front foot leaders weigh up the issues from a moral perspective of 'what is best or the right way to go'. In other words, as with all leadership perspectives, front foot thinking is a way of being, not a means of doing, an ontological rather than epistemological position.

Table 1.4 is constructed for you to score yourself. There are 26 indicators – so a top score of 260. Go for it! Such tools are useful to revisit from time to time along your leadership journey, to give feedback and remind you of such values.

Personal vision

So, what makes me a leader? Clearly, to *know* I am a leader necessitates an idea of what leadership is. The literature is resplendent with compelling descriptions: transformational, charismatic, servant, authentic, primal and suchlike. Does leadership reflect an individual's personality or is it an amalgam of traits that can be leant? Without doubt, charisma is significant. Perhaps 'presence' is a better word. Think of people who have 'presence' on the world stage.

My own inquiry explicated the following attributes:

1. Leaders are mindful; mindfulness is the hallmark of leadership.
2. Leaders are visionary (Senge 1990), with shared values congruent with its purpose.
3. Leaders are moral (Bass 1985), acting with integrity towards creating better worlds for others no matter what resistance is encountered, yet yielding graciously as appropriate.
4. Leaders have foresight (Greenleaf 2002); they are always on the front foot and anticipating the next move. Foresight is a reflection of wisdom in simply knowing what to do within a complex and largely indeterminate world.
5. Leaders are of service to enable others to accomplish what needs to be done (Greenleaf 2002) through genuine collaborative relationships that invest in people to enable them to grow and fulfil their potential.
6. Leaders are poised and emotionally intelligent in the face of disturbance and uncertainty, with the ability to sustain self within mutually supportive networks.
7. Leaders are authentic, necessarily transparent for deep trust, mindful of walking the talk of leadership, without being hooked on ego.
8. Leaders are inspirational and energetic; they lift people to higher levels of motivation and achievement within an acknowledged learning community.

Poise

The leader is poised, with the ability to know and manage self within relationships, what Goleman et al. (2002) describe as emotional intelligence (EI). Emotional intelligence is concerned with expressing and controlling emotions, both requiring a deep self-awareness guided by reflective practice. From the perspective of emotional tension the key aspects of EI are emotional self-awareness and self-control, leading to self-confidence and accurate self-assessment. The other aspects of EI relate to consequences in terms of leadership, thus providing a framework for reflection on leadership ability. The cues within the model for structured reflection nurture the development of poise.[7]

I only wanted six attributes in my leadership vision but I couldn't squeeze everything in! No doubt many more ideas could be inserted. For example, I agree with Bolman and Deal (1995) that leadership is a spiritual journey; however, there is something unsatisfactory with listing attributes. It creates an illusion that somehow we can know leadership and projects a reductionist approach whereas leadership is something whole. The risk is that it becomes an abstract model that people struggle to fit into like a suit of undersized clothing. Leadership is much more than a list of attributes. However, we do need signposts to guide us. If leadership is a whole thing, then I need a whole statement. Not an easy task given the complexity of leadership.

Tentatively I offer, 'Leadership is mindful, insightful and caring, ever vigilant of its authenticity in being of service to others within a community of practice that lifts everyone to higher levels of morality and growth, focused towards achieving shared goals and personal aspiration.'

No doubt, I could use different words. Indeed, I have played around with versions of this statement trying to find the right words to best expresses leadership. For certain, language is limiting. No matter what words you use, it is vital to reiterate that leadership is a whole thing. The eight characteristics are merely a pattern, ever changing in the light of experience and reflection and gelled through mindfulness.

My vision of leadership reflects my appreciation or appropriation of leadership ideas. The influence of theoretical ideas on my personal vision is very evident.

Scanning the web

Scanning the web for current thinking on leadership reveals many ideas that reflect the topical nature of leadership: ideas such as 'Fourteen things you should do at the start of every day'[8] (Box 1.1), 'The most successful leaders do fifteen things automatically every day'[9] (Box 1.2) and 'The seven secrets of inspiring leaders'[10] (Box 1.3). These ideas are useful to spark and stimulate the leader's curiosity and reflection –'do I do these things?' They also help make the idea of leadership fun.

Reviewing the various boxes, I must emphasise the significance of 'take a deep breath' (Box 1.1) which is the gateway to becoming present and mindful. I know this from my work as a complementary therapist working in a hospice where I take a deep breath before entering any situation in order to bring myself present to that moment. Being present is giving one's full attention to the situation having dispersed any other concerns. Being present, it then becomes possible to 'connect with others' (Box 1.1). Easier said than done. Just pause for a moment and think of how many ideas are spinning in your head at any given moment. How quickly people can let their mind be filled with a hundred things and lose control of self. Losing control creates anxiety and then the problems multiply. As Rinpoche (1992: 59) writes, 'we are fragmented into so many different aspects. We don't know who we really are, or what aspects of ourselves we should identify with or believe in. So many contradictory voices, dictates, and feelings fight for control over our inner lives that we find ourselves scattered every-where, in all directions, leaving nobody at home.'

The idea of positive energy to lift people and to serve others (Box 1.2) reflects the essential character of the leader. In serving others, the lead-er's whole perspective of power must fundamentally alter. Ideas such as lead by example, enabling others to feel safe to speak up and facilitating dialogue (Box1.2) are all powerful expressions of leadership, yet what is significant is that leaders need to be mindful of creating these moments at appropriate times, mindful of the underlying organisational culture and mindful of the potential consequences. Being mindful is being wise and compassionate – as Nelson Mandela said, having a good heart and a good head.

Box 1.1   Fourteen things you should do at the start of every day (www.forbes.com)

1	Arrive on time.
2	Take a deep breath.
3	Take five – give yourself five minutes to settle in and take a moment for yourself.
4	Start each day with a clean slate (or don't start with a hangover).
5	Don't be moody.
6	Organise your day and don't get distracted; prioritise, but be flexible.

(Continued)

7	Be present to connect with others.
8	Check in with your colleagues – sharing will enable you to achieve substantially what you need to do.
9	Ensure your workspace is organised.
10	Don't be distracted by your inbox.
11	Listen to your voicemail.
12	Place important calls and send urgent emails.
13	Take advantage of your clear head (note time of day best suited for creative exercises).
14	Plan a mid-morning break (keep the momentum going).

Box 1.2   The most successful leaders do fifteen things automatically every day

1	Make others feel safe to speak up.
2	Make expert decisions and facilitate the dialogue to empower others; focus on making things happen at all times.
3	Communicate expectations.
4	Challenge people to think.
5	Are accountable to others.
6	Lead by example.
7	Measure and reward performance (not taking others for granted).
8	Provide continuous feedback leading to reciprocal and trustworthy relationships.
9	Properly allocate and deploy talent.
10	Ask questions and seek counsel with a commitment to self-learning.
11	Problem-solve and avoid procrastination (tackle issues head on and learn from and don't avoid difficult situations).
12	Have positive energy and attitude (motivation).
13	Are great teachers (mentoring and investing in others).
14	Invest in relationships (are lifters not leaches or a loafers).
15	Genuinely enjoy responsibility – when you have reached a senior level of leadership it is about the ability to serve others and this cannot be accomplished when you do not genuinely enjoy what you do.

Box 1.3 The seven secrets of inspiring leaders (Gallo)

1	Ignite your enthusiasm.
2	Navigate a course of action (articulating a vision).
3	Sell the benefit (what's in it for me?).
4	Paint a picture (our brains are programmed more for stories than abstract ideas – stories make connections).
5	Invite participation.
6	Reinforce optimism.
7	Encourage potential (motivate and inspire your team to higher levels of achievement).

Gallo's idea of painting pictures (Box 1.3) with a focus on story encourages me, given my approach to leadership development from a story perspective through reflective practice. Stories help people see the bigger picture in ways they can connect with, particularly in relation to their own experiences or stories. As Gallo says 'stories make connections'. Throughout the book I use reflexive stories as evidence to support my own assertions on leadership.

Current leadership initiatives within the NHS

In the foreword to *Inspiring leaders: Leadership for quality initiative* (Department of Health 2009b) David Armstrong, NHS Chief Executive, writes, 'It is imperative that we align what we are doing on leadership with what we want to achieve on quality. This is what I call leadership with a purpose' (5). Armstrong aligns leadership with outcomes, for quality is generally measured in terms of outcomes not process – a view reflected in NHS leadership initiatives such as the 'Inspiring Leaders' initiative (Department of Health 2009a). It has not been my concern in this book to review the NHS leadership initiatives on offer in the UK. Each region – England, Wales, Scotland and Northern Ireland – does have different approaches which can be appreciated through web exploration. These initiatives suggest that the NHS does value leadership development although these approaches tend to fit within the dominant transactional culture that pervades the NHS and probably health care institutions worldwide.

The need for leadership development was emphasised in *Liberating the talents* (Department of Health 2002a) produced to deliver the reforms set out in the NHS plan (Department of Health 2000). It talks of effective leadership as corporate, nurturing, encouraging and inclusive, emphasising a leadership role for everyone, whatever their role, wherever they work. This language mirrors the rhetoric of transformational leadership and, in doing so, indicates a significant culture shift for an NHS built on bureaucracy, hierarchy and control. However, it does not make this shift clear, suggesting that such leadership can simply be accommodated within normal organisational patterns.

The NHS Leadership Academy's leadership model states (http://www.leadershipacademy.nhs.uk):

The Healthcare Leadership Model has been developed to help staff who work in health and care to become better leaders. It is useful for everyone – whether you have a formal leadership responsibility or not, if you work in a clinical or other service setting and if you work with a team of five people or 5,000. It describes the things you can see leaders doing at work, and is organised in a way that helps everyone to see how they can develop as a leader. It applies equally to a whole variety of roles and settings that exist within health and care. We want to help you understand how your leadership behaviours affect the culture and climate you, your colleagues and teams work in. Whether you work directly with patients and service users or not, you will realise what you do and how you behave will affect the experiences of patients and service users of your organisation, the quality of care provided and the reputation of the organisation itself.

The health care leadership model consists of nine 'leadership dimensions' (Table 1.5). In the second dimension the model states: 'Having the essential personal qualities for leaders'. The model further notes,

The way that we manage ourselves is a central part of being an effective leader. It is vital to recognise that personal qualities like self-awareness, self-confidence, self-control, self-knowledge, personal reflection, resilience and determination are the foundation of how we behave. Being aware of your strengths and limitations in these areas will have a direct effect on how you behave and interact with others, and they with you. Without this awareness, it will be much more difficult (if not impossible) to behave in the way research has shown that leaders should. This, in turn, will have a direct impact on your colleagues, any team you work in, and the overall culture and climate within the team as well as within the organisation. Whether you work directly with patients and service users or not, this can affect the care experience they have. Working positively on these personal qualities will lead to a focus on care and high-quality services for patients and service users, their carers and their families.

	What is it?
Inspiring shared purpose	Valuing a service ethos; curious about how to improve services and patient care; behaving in a way that reflects the principles and values of the NHS
Leading with care	Having the essential personal qualities for leaders in health and social care; understanding the unique qualities and needs of a team; providing a caring, safe environment to enable everyone to do their jobs effectively
Evaluating information	Seeking out varied information; using information to generate new ideas and make effective plans for improvement or change; making evidence-based decisions that respect different perspectives and meet the needs of all service users
Connecting our services	Understanding how health and social care services fit together and how different people, teams or organisations interconnect and interact
Sharing the vision	Communicating a compelling and credible vision of the future in a way that makes it feel achievable and exciting
Engaging the team	Involving individuals and demonstrating that their contributions and ideas are valued and important for delivering outcomes and continuous improvements to the service
Holding to account	Agreeing clear performance goals and quality indicators; supporting individuals and teams to take responsibility for results; providing balanced feedback
Developing capability	Building capability to enable people to meet future challenges; using a range of experiences as a vehicle for individual and organisational learning; acting as a role model for personal development
Influencing for results	Deciding how to have a positive impact on other people; building relationships to recognise other people's passions and concerns; using interpersonal and organisational understanding to persuade and build collaboration

Table 1.5 Nine dimensions of the health care leadership model

It is these personal qualities, notably *self-awareness and personal reflection*, that I believe are most significant, because without this awareness it will be impossible to become a leader. Personal reflection is the key to developing self-awareness. It is this awareness that ultimately cultures mindfulness.

However, the leader faces another significant challenge to becoming a leader, that of the transactional culture that characterises health care organisations. Hence there is a tension between the idea of leadership and realising its reality in a culture that despite espousing the rhetoric of leadership is antipathetic to it simply because true leadership demands an organisational revolution from the top-down. People are so locked in their unreflective ways that change becomes difficult, wrapped up as they are in bureaucratic hierarchical power relationships and egos. The idea of 'lead by example' must ultimately stem from the top down; otherwise aspiring leaders will bang their heads against the hard transactional wall. Without doubt, becoming a true leader is not easy. Understanding and resolving this tension so that the vision of leadership becomes realised is the primary focus of reflective practice.

The desire for genuine leadership shines through the 'Inspiring Leaders' paper, yet change fundamentally hinges on the level of existence – can the transactional world radically shift or simply accommodate the idea of leadership to fit into its transactional world? Many leaders are in managerial positions. Rodriguez (1995) describes managers as people who prefer control, stability and exert power through such means as task orientation and quantitative styles. The risk is that the transactional approach becomes more determined and perhaps more ruthless in meeting quality outcomes at a time of severe economic restraint. I am not optimistic. It is not difficult to see that when external agencies set budgets and award stars for good performance against imposed outcome measures, the gaze of management turns towards reaching those outcomes. Leaders emphasise the process, not the product. Loori (2004: 93–4) writes, 'When we try and reach a goal, we become fixated on it and we miss the process. Process and goal are the same reality. Each step clearly contains the goal.'

It's not difficult to realise that if staff are respected and valued and feel involved then they will perform better: work harder, put in the extra effort when necessary, take more responsibility and use their initiative, have higher motivation, and be happier and less stressed. You do not need statistical evidence to make this point. Just open your minds. Put like this, you must wonder at the failure of organisations to invest in effective leadership development. I do not mean two- or three-day workshops, such as the Leading Empowered Organisations (LEO)[11] programme, that barely scratch the surface of leadership yet create illusions of leadership investment.

Della, a deputy director of nursing, writes: The Leading Empowered Organisations (LEO) training promises to provide nurses with the skills they need to be effective leaders and to challenge status quo within health care, by supporting staff at all levels to lead and effect change in organisations and providing a basis for developing healthy relationships, skilled problem solving and confident risk taking. On the basis of understanding that leadership skills cannot be taught (Senge 1990) and certainly cannot be developed on a three-day course, my reader should not be surprised to learn that personal experience of LEO training (delivered by senior nurses who are considered to be 'leading lights' within today's NHS in England) is not entirely positive. Taking three days out of practice was beneficial in enabling me to stand back and reflect on my role as leader; however, most of the material used was already familiar to me, having being exposed to it via previous senior management training. Not surprisingly, the focus of training was not inquiry as the literature suggests but on problem solving and advocacy skills concerned predominantly with meeting predetermined national course objectives, namely:

- Supporting nurses to challenge authority
- Enabling nurses to accept responsibility for reducing levels of administration and bureaucracy by challenging the status quo
- Encouraging nurses to challenge misuse of resources
- Encouraging nurses to influence change in front-line services
- Enabling nurses to improve access to services

The course content focused around these topics was delivered via a workbook with pre-prepared questions and answers in order to maintain consistent message delivery across England. Only now can I comment on the absence of learner input and flexibility, as I have come to appreciate how stability, structure and sameness (Porter O'Grady 1992) are the basis of the teaching and how, from this, culturally induced behaviours are likely to reflect the course values and perceptions when and if implemented into practice. Cynically, I use the metaphor of nurses as robots and question the hidden agenda that lies behind this leadership package.

Freire writes (1972: 23), 'One of the basic elements of a relationship between oppressor and oppressed is prescription.' I now consider the imposition of this teaching. For the majority of the thousands of nurses who have accessed this training, like myself, it would have been 'sold' as a liberating opportunity, as indeed I have ignorantly sold it to others, and as such, being chosen to attend is in itself a privilege.

Kelly writes: As well as having a nurse practitioner role, I had been elected by my colleagues to serve as the board nurse member for a local Primary Care Group (PCG). Like those who elected me, I believed that my extensive knowledge of primary care and willingness to speak out were the qualities to lead changes in the way services were delivered. However, it soon became clear to me that leadership was much more than willingness to have a voice. Reflecting back on those PCG meetings I can now see how ill-prepared my nurse colleagues and I were for this important role. This became evident with the new agenda for nurse executives that required us to engage with staff and lead changes. Without adequate training and understanding of the skills required, many PCG nurse members struggled to engage and lead (Wilkin et al. 2001).

Repeated requests for help from the PCG management team resulted in several workshops around leading and managing. The PCG management team, like the nurses, were of the opinion that leadership could be taught. Although the workshops were very interesting and gave us insight into project management, communication and leading change, none of them ever addressed the personal qualities needed for leadership. There was a general belief that anyone who used the techniques outlined in the training would become a good leader.

As a nurse executive member I was immediately enrolled on the Leading Empowered Organisations (LEO) course, which was one of the Department of Health courses that was to create nurse leaders in three days. The course was to create empowered and visionary nurses who would be valued and nurtured towards becoming effective leaders (Faugier and Woolnough 2003). However, in reality, all it achieved was frustrated staff who felt empowered but became demoralised when they returned to the work place and realised how little control they actually could achieve (Rippon 2001). This was evident in my own role as a nurse executive member where despite my senior position I found my ideas blocked and my enthusiasm for change dampened by more senior nurse managers in the organisation. I began to question why I was experiencing such difficulties in bringing about change. Was it because I lacked effective leadership skills? Or was it because those in more senior positions also lacked effective leadership skills and were unable to cope with this new way of working? After all, many nurse managers have traditionally evolved into these roles and were somehow expected to develop leadership

(Continued)

skills along the way. Critchley (2001) supports this view, stating that there is a false assumption that those in senior positions are already effective leaders by virtue of their status in the organisation. It soon became clear to me that their defensive behaviour may have been due to their own lack of leadership. Although the LEO course had made me more aware of the need to develop personal leadership skills, it also made me realise how little influence I had within the NHS. Faugier and Woolnough (2003) identified that this was a common feeling amongst senior nurses who reported feeling like a 'cog in the wheel of a very large organisation' (25). Many of them described leadership within their organisations as driven by senior managers to establish order and control.

For the first time since becoming a nurse over twenty years ago, I began to question my own style of leadership. I always believed I was a natural leader as all through my life I had taken leading roles. At school I was always games captain, the elected student lead, and in my nursing career I had quickly progressed to becoming a ward sister.

Without question I would have described myself as a leader, someone who had never flinched from responsibility and was always willing to stand up and be counted. But did this make me a leader or just someone who likes to be in control? Kerfoot (2002) suggests that the old style of command and control has been a strong component of leadership within the culture of nursing for many years. It was uncomfortable to think of myself as a controller but the more I reflected on this issue, the more I became aware of times when indeed I had controlled situations. I justified my actions by a need to ensure that patients received the best possible care. After all I had come into nursing with the desire to care for others, and I was willing to put everything into achieving the highest standards of care. Delivering a quality standard of care was something I took pride in.

Taking some control and managing other staff was something that I had thought was part of the role of a senior nurse, and although it was always carried out politely there was little real thought for my colleagues. Sofarelli and Brown (1998) would suggest these are the actions of a manager concerned with achieving outcomes to meet service needs. Although I was not employed as a manager there was an element of management within my workload that of course required me to meet organisational goals. Looking back, I am aware

(Continued)

that I was occasionally so focused on meeting the goals of the organisation that I had encouraged and directed others to go along with my plans without really understanding their needs. This again stems from my competitive nature of achieving goals effectively and not being seen to fail. Covey (2002) suggests that this is poor leadership, as concern for the people you manage tends to become less important than meeting organisational targets.

The more I questioned myself, the more I realised that leadership was much more than just pushing staff in the right direction. The LEO course had been sparse in its content but it did make me question my view of leadership. I spent time trying to work out what made individuals good at leadership. I thought about those individuals I had worked with who had taken leading roles such as ward sisters and departmental managers. There had been a mixture of good and poor leaders, but the odd few had stood out in memory as exceptional leaders and people I had enjoyed working with. I began to reflect on what bit it was about those individuals that had made such an impression on me. They were all different people with different ways of working but the key thing that stood out was how they made me feel valued and empowered.

Conclusion

I have surveyed some ideas on leadership that inspire the aspiring leaders to create a vision of leadership. Of course, these are only some ideas. I expect readers will google leadership to reveal an extensive literature and deepen their theoretical sources to inform their leadership journeys.

Reflection

- Write your personal vision of leadership. You may wish to complete reading the book and return to this exercise. You may want to explore leadership literature more widely and deeply to be better informed.
- Share your vision with colleagues. How do they react?
- Consider how this vision can become a reality? What obviously constrains me?

Notes

1. See Appendix A1 for details of the 'Influences grid' within the Model for Structured Reflection.
2. Rebecca alludes to types of power, following French and Raven (see Figure 5.3).
3. I term this dialogue between theory and practice as known through reflection as the third dialogical movement of narrative construction. See Appendix 2.
4. The MSc Health Care Leadership programme module 'Alternative perspectives on leadership assignment' – the leaders were required to shadow and observe leaders in practice. Many of the leaders asked these leaders to score themselves against used Schuster's ten attributes of transformational leadership. These leaders scored themselves as transformational on every attribute except two – 'you share power with others' and 'you risk, experiment and learn' (see Figure 3.1). See also Appendix 1 for programme outline.
5. See Figure 5.3.
6. See Department of Health guidance paper – *A consultation on strengthening the NHS constitution* published in November 2012. The paper noted that the main changes proposed include a 'new responsibility for staff to treat patients not only with the highest standards of care, but also with compassion, dignity and respect'.
7. See Appendix 1 figure.
8. http://www.forbes.com/pictures/efjd45ekmj/14-things-you-should-do-at-the-start-of-every-work-day/ (Accessed 10 October 2014).
9. http://www.forbes.com/sites/glennllopis/2013/02/18/the-most-successful-leaders-do-15-things-automatically-every-day/ (Accessed 10 October 2014).
10. www.forbes.com/sites/carminegallo/2011/07/06/the-7-secrets-of-inspiring-leaders/ (Accessed 9 October 2014).
11. Leading an empowered organisation programme. See *Developing excellence in leadership within urgent care: Tomorrow's nurse leaders today* (Department of Health (2003)). It states, 'Developing leadership is an integral part of the Government's Modernisation Agenda and the NHS Plan. Effective leadership is crucial for improving the quality of care for patients, for developing staff and for creating the vision to take the modernisation agenda forward.'

2 The Adventure Has Only Just Begun!

Introduction

Narrative is a powerful method of communicating ideas because it paints a big picture that is both contextual and subjective. It enables the reader to feel the issues being explored and relate to them in terms of her own experiences. In this way, narrative opens a dialogical learning space. So, as you read, ask yourself, 'How do I relate to this?'

Martha writes: My journey of becoming a leader is an adventure story. The idea of an adventure conjures up images of exploring new and unpredictable terrains. As with any gripping adventure story there are situations of failure and success along the way. At the beginning, I truly believed I knew my plans for my professional future. I had been a qualified nurse for four years and had progressed rapidly through the ranks to become a senior nurse in the strategic post of National Service Framework for the Older Person Co-ordinator at a medium-sized acute NHS trust. I had career aspirations that would take me to the highest and most satisfying level in the organisational hierarchy where I would realise my full potential and become all that I could be. I have always been ambitious, stemming from my childhood where performing well at school was highly prized and rewarded. Success in any activity was the desired goal and motivator. I grew up in a family that lived by a very strong moral code largely as a result of strict religious convictions and beliefs that continue to influence me today.

My career aspirations led me to believe that a further academic qualification was necessary if I was to successfully achieve my goal and indeed this was the professional advice proffered by my organisation. Much of my previous learning had been concerned with goal achievement and attainment with a focus on specific subjects and outcomes (Houle 1961). The learning process had invariably ceased on successful completion of the course attended and the certificate awarded – the end product had, to my mind, been achieved.

I commenced the leadership programme from this orientation of learning with a very limited perception of the opportunities it would present.

Reality shock, yet I quickly adapted and became alive to the possibilities that this course would offer me in terms of self-perception and development. I was forced to come face to face with myself – an experience that on occasions I found disturbing – yet it led to the discovery of a new, far more satisfying way of learning and a set of new horizons and vistas to explore. My learning quickly became oriented to the learning process itself and I developed a genuine interest in the subject of leadership. The original goal of academic achievement became subsumed in my new commitment to learning and leadership development far beyond the completion of the course.

I commenced the course as a diehard, almost evangelistic, theorist. I had previously studied the four learning styles of Honey and Mumford (1989) and recognised that my preference was always for logically sound theories that fitted into rational schemes. As a theorist I readily accepted, usually without question, basic assumptions, principles, theories and models and preferred rational objectivity rather than anything subjective or ambiguous. I often rejected the other learning styles of activism, pragmatism and reflection and they were not really part of my psyche. I had paid scant attention to them in the past only utlising them where necessary to fulfil the requirements of academic courses attended. My theoretical stance was probably based on my strong adherence to the notion of evidence-based practice, that is 'doing the right things right' – a belief so strongly felt that I was chair of the evidence-based practice council for my organisation (Muir Gray 1997). Evidence-based practice has arguably become the 'buzz word' of health care. It had been a foremost element in the linguistic currency of my nurse training and is a pervasive element in the clinical governance agenda so widely espoused in my organisation. The UK government's drive to modernise health care includes a commitment to the provision of health services based on evidence, and published strategies for nursing emphasise the need for a robust evidence base (Department of Health 1997, 1999). I saw this need for evidence as a basis for effective practice as paramount, that for me, meant adherence to objective and proven theory. I felt comfortable with this concept possibly because, as Craig and Smyth (2002) note, evidence-based practice is a phrase that trips lightly off the tongue, engenders a reassuring glow that all is well and signifies that nurses merely need to implement the available evidence. As the course developed, I recognised that 'evidence-based practice' is one of the most used but least understood ideas in health care. Nursing (and nurse leadership) rarely lends itself to the application of research evidence and technical rationality (Schön 1987). This course was about to radically question my mode of thinking and learning style and open doors into other ways of thinking and perception. This new way of thinking was particularly exciting to me and I became acutely aware that such a strong and rigid adherence to the notion that evidence can provide all of the answers brings with it the danger of stifling creativity (Johns 2004a).

Navone (1977) reminds me that all stories begin with the word 'And' since there is always something that precedes every experience; in this case the accumulated effects of many years of life, formative influences and career aspirations for the future. My life history is not a liability to be exorcised but is the very precondition for knowing (Pinar 1981). Rogers (1998) writes that new students are not new people – rather they possess a set of values, established prejudices and attitudes in which they have a great deal of emotional investment all based on past experiences. Undertaking the leadership programme enabled me to test some of these life influences and more fully appreciate their meaning and validity. It has given me a better understanding of my true self and in a sense has given me control over who I am. I commenced the course then as an outcome-focused practitioner with a rigid set of ideas and beliefs, but with no concept of the literally life-changing leadership opportunities that were about to present.

Beginning to lead myself

I must first illuminate the significant events that occurred in the first months of the course that enabled me to appreciate my mindset when I took my first steps on this leadership adventure. The first months were a time of deepening anxieties in my professional life that ultimately led to my taking a truly emancipatory step. I had felt increasingly dissatisfied with my role as National Service Framework for Older Person Co-ordinator for the trust. The role felt like a 'political' appointment to fulfil the trust's requirement to comply with the national standards. Financial resources were not available to make the necessary significant changes in practice, and my direct line manager was an extremely transactional operator who had begun to make attempts to change my job profile in a way that I felt was unacceptable. One particular experience early in the course proved to be the decisive event that gave me the opportunity to closely reflect upon my role at that time and the deep disquiet I felt within.

In my journal I write:

> June 2002 – I had a meeting with Eve from the clinical governance unit today and I can't believe what has happened. On our returns to the Royal College of Physicians stroke audit the trust has declared that we have a stroke unit as required by the NSF [National Service Framework]. Well, we don't! All we have is a bay on a medical ward that stroke patients go

to if they're lucky enough to get a bed! How does that constitute a stroke unit? It has no specialist staff, no recognised or co-ordinated extended stroke team and no equipment. Eve is just as concerned about this mis-representation as I am and I feel implicated in this without my choosing. I feel decidedly uneasy – why be so disingenuous to say we have something when we don't? I suppose it will be said that it's all down to interpretation and that we must be seen to meet the standard. I can't help feeling this is all wrong and I wonder if I want to be a part of all this anymore?

I knew that continuation in my role as it was would culminate in a personal crisis or that I may surrender and become comfortably numb about the whole role expectation. Inspired by the leadership course I felt empowered to quit. I write in my journal:

> July 2002 – Well I told A today that I was leaving. She seemed very inter-ested at first but as soon as I told her I was going back to the clinical area to be a ward sister her attitude changed. She seems to think it's a bad career move as it's a lower grade but I know it's right for me. I want to be somewhere where I have real influence over what happens to patients and colleagues not just in a 'tick box' job. I suppose it's the old attitude that clinical work is of lower status than a managerial job. In a final transac-tional comment she actually said that I couldn't be released from my post for two months and I had to remind her that my contract allowed me to give only four weeks notice! I don't feel that I failed in that job because on this occasion I have accepted that there are some things I cannot change and perhaps the best move is to distance myself from it all and to start somewhere new where I can be a force for good. I actually feel totally emancipated and am looking forward to the future 'back on the ward'.

I no longer felt that the higher-graded roles were the pinnacle of achieve-ment. The scene was set for my leadership journey. A line had been drawn under the unsatisfactory past and I stepped into my new role as ward sister and leader of the ward team with an acute awareness of self and an enthu-siasm that had long been missing from my practice.

Leading the ward team

The ward team is in turmoil. Morale low. In my journal I write

> August 2003 – What a bad day! Everyone on the ward seems to be fighting with everyone else at the moment. I think they're all tired and overworked because of the hot weather combined with severe staff

shortages and pressures of work. The health care assistants are at each other's throats arguing over who is doing the most work, staff sickness rates are soaring, the trained staff are arguing with the health care assistants and are criticising each other, the students seem particularly difficult to manage, the hospital is sweltering and I'm stuck in the middle of it all. There is no productive discussion going on about anything at the moment, no one seems happy and the team really is on the road to self-destruction! The ward manager seems ineffectual in sorting this out so perhaps it's down to me to be the proactive one. I simply can't go along with her avoidance of it – I really need to think about how and why it's all gone wrong and what I (we as a team) can do to put it right.

Avoidance of the problem is not an option if I am going to fulfil my leadership role. After one particularly angst-riddled day I was determined to discover the reasons why the team had become so discordant over the previous few months and use the transformational leadership model as a means to develop and sustain an effective team ward.

Tuning into the voices of the shadow system revealed to me the reasons for the team's discordance. Lindberg et al. (1998) note that everyone in an organisation belongs to two systems: the legitimate and the shadow. The legitimate system consists of formal hierarchy, rules and communication patterns, while the shadow system lies behind the scenes and consists of the hallway conversation, the grapevine, the rumour mill and the informal procedures for getting things done. Membership of the shadow system contributes significantly to people's mental models and subsequent action and seems therefore a critical feature in understanding the workings of the clinical environment. Learning about the shadow system enabled me to see that I had unwittingly tapped into it without really understanding the significance of its existence at that time. It became clear that the team often felt overwhelmed by their work demands. They believed they had little control or influence in their working environment and received little or no support from managers. Olofsson et al. (2003) describe these as critical factors that promote negative stress in the work environment. These negative stressors had, I believed, resulted in an explosion of 'horizontal violence', a well-known phenomenon where inter-group conflict occurs as a way of releasing tension when the group feels unable to direct its aggression at the perceived oppressor (the organisation and its managers) (Farrell 2001). While people are clearly the most important resource in any organisation and therefore should command a great deal of attention from management, this attention is frequently missing (Farrell 2001). This seemed the case here, and I observed that although she was aware of the turbulence on the ward, the ward manager consistently avoided it. In response, I suggested a team 'away day' for all nursing staff as a means to come together and engage in dialogue. Interestingly, the ward manager declined to attend, although she was happy for me to facilitate the day. I sensed she was threatened by such an opportunity for staff to express themselves freely. Mindful of the notion that I did not have to confront all problems at once, I decided that was an issue for later action. My approach to the 'away day' was inspired by the idea of the learning organisation (LO), 'where people continually expand their capacities to create the results they truly desire, where new and expansive patterns of thinking are nurtured, where collective aspiration is set free, and where people are continually learning how to learn together' (Senge 1990: 3).

I intentionally used dialogue, in contrast to discussion, to facilitate the staff to explore why the ward was infected with such low morale. Talk about opening a can of worms! We did not solve all problems but the dialogue helped the team to develop strategies to articulate and recognise the stressors. Verbal feedback from the 'away day' participants was positive but I felt quite saddened by the comments such as 'No one had listened to us before today', and 'We've never all been allowed off the ward to talk together in this way before'. I sense the way the organisation is worried by what it may hear or that the views of its staff are considered unimportant. Subsequent experiences were to illuminate these thoughts further. Ending the day on a positive note, my journal entry reveals my feelings.

August 2003 – What a relief! I was worried about what I might be writing tonight but I think the away day today went really well. I felt it was a huge risk as I haven't tried anything like it before and I guess it could have all gone wrong and ended up as a moaning and groaning session. On a positive note, there was a lot of 'dialogue' and I think we managed to bring some sensitive issues out into the open at last. I was surprised how easy it was to get people to talk and to sometimes voluntarily surface their feelings, thoughts and acceptance of the consequences of their behaviours with no prompting from me. Had things become difficult I would have had to engage in some fairly rapid reflection in action to resolve the situation. Could I have coped with that? – I don't know. Having had this experience though I feel better prepared for the next time. Perhaps I underestimated the propensity of the team to engage in such a positive way. A thought for me in the future – be more confident and optimistic about the abilities of others and stop being so paternalistic! Perhaps that is a remnant of my transactional thinking there? It was a good idea for us all to have lunch together afterwards – people were actually talking and laughing socially again, something that had somehow been lost along the way.

Following the away day, I reflected on whether I had demonstrated any of Schuster's (1994) twelve leadership capacities each of which is under-pinned by deep thinking (head), empathy (heart) and congruent action (hand), (Schuster's attributes of leadership). I chose Schuster as my lead-ership theory template because firstly, it is grounded in transformational leadership ideals, and secondly it made sense. Perhaps I found Schuster easy to identify with because of its checklist nature. Schuster cautions against viewing these attributes as a simple list as this would inevitably lead to a reductionist and instrumental approach where each attribute is viewed as a task to be accomplished. He acknowledges that leadership is much greater than the sum of these parts. The list is like pointing to the moon. My dif-ficulty with Schuster, as I assume with all leadership theory, is appreciating what these values mean as lived rather than as words written on paper. Schuster asserts that leaders, whilst holding their own vision of practice, are carful not to impose these on followers. Rather, the leader facilitates a collaborative vision, influencing it as appropriate to ensure it offers a stimu-lating and intellectual path to practice.

Of course, empathy is the hallmark of nursing – for how can a nurse respond to a patient if she is unable to connect with that patient's experi-ence and meanings of illness? In much the same way, how can a leader connect with her followers if she does not appreciate their experience? Schuster acknowledges the significance of action aligning with words; it is one thing to talk fine words but another to genuinely live them. The ego is wrapped up in self-concern and protecting self from anxiety. Hence in a high-anxiety organisation, then people inevitably become absorbed in self. As such, knowing and accepting self is a major focus for my leadership devel-opment. Moving down the attributes I could continue this commentary, but they are generally self-explanatory. However, it is worthy to emphasise that leadership embraces administration to counter any idea that leadership and management are separate. I feel my ward sister role becomes increasingly bureaucratic! I am sure most ward sisters or managers would agree. Paper-work piles up! I am in a management role and I must manage through the qualities of leadership, concerned with human relationships and growth, yet still mindful of organisational aims.

Schuster's attributes of leadership:

- You hold a vision for the organisation that is intellectually rich, stimulat-ing and rings true.
- You are honest and empathetic. People feel emotionally safe and trust that you have their interests at heart.
- Your character is well-developed, without the prominent dark side of ego power – your behaviour aligns with your words.

- You set aside your own interests in looking good and getting strokes instead making others look good and giving others power and credit.
- You evince a concern for the whole (not just your organisation) reflected in your passionate and ethical voice being heard when necessary.
- Your natural tendency is to develop others to become engaged, deepen perspectives and be effective.
- You can share power with others – you believe sharing power is the best way to tap talent, engage others and get work done in optimal fashion.
- You risk, experiment and learn. Information is never complete.
- You have a true passion for work and the vision that is evident in commitment of time, attention to detail and ability to renew your energy.
- You effectively communicate, both listening and speaking.
- You understand and appreciate management and administration. They appreciate that; you move towards shared success without sacrifice.
- You celebrate the now. At meetings or wherever, you sincerely acknowledge accomplishment, staying in the moment before moving on.
- You persist in hard times. That means you have the courage to move ahead when you're tired, conflicted and getting mixed signals.

Through *effective communication, both listening and speaking*, I had shared my personal vision for the ward. The team had then come to a mutual agreement about what our *shared* vision should be. While *acknowledging our accomplishments* as a team to date, I had been *honest and empathetic* about the current difficulties the team faced.

Without behaving in an overtly transactional style, I had introduced the necessity of a certain standard of behaviour while inviting those present to offer their thoughts and feelings to the group. This involved some *risk taking and experimentation* since the outcome of such an invitation is unpredictable. We had engaged in dialogue where all had been encouraged to share experiences and thoughts on an equal footing. While facilitating the day I had not clung to a timed agenda but rather had *shared power* with the group, following issues as they arose.

Although I had initially been anxious about adopting this approach, I felt comfortable with my new approach and excited by the challenges and opportunities it presented. I also felt strangely rebellious, as this approach was anathema to my organisation, but revelled in this new sensation and was intensely motivated by the positive outcome of the 'away day'. I had previously chaired groups in a transactional manner in accordance with organisational tradition where formal agendas to achieve organisational goals and strict control of the participants were viewed as signs of a good chair. Now, I knew a different way. Perhaps responding in a transformational manner was easier for me since the staff did not know me and had no experience of my transactional history! Yet did they trust me? Perhaps this was all superficial?

In the subsequent months, it became clear that the 'away day' was successful in restoring the usually harmonious relationship among the ward nursing team. By common consensus, the ward became a much more positive place to work. The seeds of trust had been sown and it was vital I did not compromise this trust. Collaborative conflict management style and facilitation of dialogue, both during arranged meetings and informally, became new norms. We began work on constructing a shared vision to replace the tattered old copy I found buried in the desk drawer and which had no relevance to everyday practice written as it was in corporate speak.

Persisting in hard times

How easily trust can shatter! My current ward was one of two wards within the orthopaedic directorate designated as an elective surgery plus trauma area, each with its own sister but sharing a manager. The other ward was permanently closed at extremely short notice and with no discussion with any of the staff working there. My journal demonstrates the frenzy of emotions that I felt:

> August 2003 – I cannot believe what has happened today. June (the other ward sister) and I were called into the manager's office at 1 p.m. and told the news. It was a complete and utter shock to us both. It had been decided at very senior level and was presented as a fait accompli – no discussion! June was very upset particularly when she was told that her staff would be offered other jobs dispersed around the hospital. Ward closure hadn't been discussed at all with the ward sisters and now we were being told to tell the staff. I don't think June or I was thinking straight – we had no time to let the news sink in and the next shift was about to start. We were told that the staff had to know now about the closure as the new ward occupiers (urology) were coming to look around their new area in half an hour. The manager didn't even suggest that she do the job herself and didn't even come out of the office and on to the ward. June and I went straight back to the ward area and told the staff who were very upset and angry – lots of tears all around. Some of these girls had worked with each other for fifteen years and of course they are all worried about their jobs now. Lots of recriminations – why is it June's ward that is closing and not mine? I don't know the answer to this but I think the next two weeks will be very difficult. I am so angry at the organisation's transactional behaviour – riding roughshod over the

staff with no seeming concern for their feelings – just the needs of the organisation. Some of the staff were angry with June and me, insisting that as we were the ward sisters, we must have known about this so why didn't we tell them?

I felt an intense cacophony of emotions. This incident really brought home to me the challenge of being a transformational leader within the transactional organisation. My leadership skills were strained and challenged as I tried to keep true to my leadership path. The week that followed this entry was particularly difficult. June and I became the 'victims' of a great deal of horizontal violence, as staff, who felt completely powerless in the face of considerable change imposed from above, vented their anger at us and each other. I was well aware that the 'shadow system', as a result of the sudden change, regarded June and me with some suspicion as part of an elite group privy to information that we did not actually have. Marris (1986) describes this as a tribal response to crisis. The change had been badly managed from those in high authority in a power-coercive way (Bennis et al. 1984) with no attempt to include staff involvement – a strategy unlikely to win over the hearts and minds of those caught up in the change (Sheehan 1990). The organisation's pervasive insensitivity to the staff betrayed an indifference to their feelings. There was no recognition of the loss experienced by the staff and their sense of personal confusion of identity, provoked by the inevitable disruption in working relationships and working patterns.

Throughout this period, I found the leadership road hard to travel. It was difficult to be transformational in the face of a barrage of suspicion and criticism and there were times when I felt completely inept in the face of the organisation's enormous power. I felt that, as nurses, we had all been deemed unworthy of consultation about the change although we were probably the ones to be most affected by it. Even the senior nurse in the unit, the modern matron, denied that she had been consulted, which raised significant questions from the ward staff about her role. Despite all the rhetoric, it seemed that matron's power sadly was more symbolic than functional with the consequence that her role may indeed have been created merely to satisfy the whim of politicians, doctors and managers (Kitching 1993, Watson and Thompson 2003).

The ward manager and matron withdrew to their offices – a classically non-productive avoidance response to any kind of conflict from managers ill-prepared to deal with stress (Valentine 1994, Whetten et al. 1996). I felt very exposed. It was hard to manage the change in a positive manner once it had been imposed, although I did suspect that the bed reconfiguration might be beneficial to the organisation in the long run. It was not the change itself that I found objectionable but the way it had been forced upon the staff. The greatest challenge for me during this whole period was the need to manage the anger I felt towards the organisation and to the members of staff who had wrongly assumed my alignment and agreement with the organisation's transactional approach.

This was a time when I had to daily 'prove' my transformational leadership by my leadership behaviour. I was determined to ensure my behaviour constantly aligned with my leadership values. Leaders who practise what they preach enhance their credibility and competence and become the leaders who succeed (Freemantle 1992). By consistently demonstrating concern for the staff, maintaining open lines of communication, discussing employment moves, providing psychological support where necessary and helping with the physical practicalities of ward closure, the staff came to regard me as a credible leader who did understand and appreciate their concerns. Some of them expressed surprise that I had no hesitation in verbalising criticism regarding the organisation's management of the change as though it was the norm that ward sisters should unquestioningly fall in line with any organisational objective, whatever that may be! *Persistence in hard times* paid off and by the time of the ward closure, I felt that my credibility as a transformational leader had been restored. While I am perhaps alone unable to take on all the might of the larger organisation, I considered that my transformational behaviours at least mitigated against the more damaging impact for staff – as one of my colleagues noted, 'You helped to soften the blow.'

In my journal I write:

> September 2003 – Well, the last day for June's ward. The party went well and there were cakes and flowers and lots of friendly hugging. People were tearful but resigned now to the change. The ward manager didn't appear at the party and when I saw her and asked if she was going she just said that she didn't like all that emotional stuff! Surely, had she been a true leader, her role would have been seen as pivotal in the ward set-up but it seems that, at the end, she ignored the staff and they ignored her. Perhaps such emotional detachment is the mark of a truly consummate transactional leader.

The whole experience had really brought home to me the transactional culture of the organisation. I was part of it! As ward sister, it seems that other staff may view me, particularly those who do not know me well, as just a willing cog in the controlling organisation. I often sense that my organisation finds me irritating, an all-too-obvious flaw in their transactional, controlling veneer. It took courage to challenge an organisation when it seems I am the lone voice in a sea of such transactional proportions.

Person-centred leadership

Being a transformational leader within the transactional organisation that expects its managers and ward sisters to behave in a controlling, authoritative and regulatory manner towards staff members is not easy. The performance management procedures and the organisation's policy for their expected 'core behaviours' from staff do not sit comfortably with my desire to establish collaborative relationships with staff. Such transactional practices seem to have little regard for those persons working within the organisation but simply serve to ensure that the organisation produces its goods and services efficiently and that it serves the needs of those persons who control it (Mintzberg 1973).

My leadership of the individual was challenged and tested by an incident when a newly qualified staff nurse made a serious drug error. The organisation's response was to place her on a performance development plan. This plan was written by senior management and handed to me to implement.

I journal:

> October 2003 – Today I was handed a performance management plan for Claire by the ward manager. Claire has apparently made a serious drug error and I am expected to 'supervise' and 'monitor' her progress through this plan to ensure her 'competence' to practise. Poor Claire came into the office to see me – shaking and upset. She seemed absolutely terrified about the plan and what it involved and was obviously deeply upset by what had happened. I immediately felt that this was not the way I would like to handle the issue. As a fellow nurse I did not want to see a colleague so distraught nor did I want to be cast in the role of dictatorial manager against my will. Claire and I talked briefly – I assured her that I did not consider her to be 'in trouble' as she put it but rather that we would work through the problem together. We arranged to meet tomorrow. Today was very busy and I want to give Claire the time we need to discuss where we go from here. It also gives me time to think how to handle this! Claire left the office a little less upset but clearly worried. I need to handle this very carefully – she is very vulnerable and I'm concerned that this will really knock her confidence.

This journal entry signified quite a change in my approach. Almost to my shame, I am aware that prior to this course, I would probably willingly have endorsed such a plan as a means to 'protect the public'. Any concern for Claire would be minimal and my priority would have been to fulfil the highly transactional, retributive role expected of me. In a complete turnaround, my immediate response to this incident was to consider whether I should refuse to be responsible for such a transactional performance development plan. However, I quickly dismissed this suggestion as a mere avoidance tactic and in the full knowledge that if I did not implement the plan then someone else undoubtedly would. I knew this would not help Claire but rather would be an abdication of my leadership responsibility.

The plan was in my hands and so I began to consider how I could turn around a transactional 'order' into a developmental opportunity for Claire. I needed to recognise the potential harm to the patient of the drug error but dealing with this aspect only required the thinking (head) aspect of leadership. To be a truly transformational leader, I needed to utilise the empathy (heart) aspect of leadership to help Claire learn and grow. Schuster (1994) notes that both head (thinking) and heart (empathy) are both essential capacities of the transformational leader but that heart is the more difficult of the two aspects to develop. Perhaps this is why most organisations ignore this aspect of leadership and concentrate more fully on the thinking required to exert power and control.

Drawing on previous experience, I considered the way clinical supervision[1] could be useful to support and guide Claire through the learning process. I sensed that Claire might view the process of clinical supervision as a hostile, pseudo-analytic process of belittlement, criticism, shaming and attribution of blame (Cottrell 1999). Johns (2001) distinguishes between emancipatory and technical supervision that mirrors the difference between transformational and transactional cultures. In emancipatory supervision, the supervisor enables the practitioner to negotiate her own growth agenda, whereas, in technical supervision, it is the supervisor who sets the agenda according to organisation goals. The contrast is stark, yet helpful for me to realise that, as a transformational leader, I *must* respond from an emancipatory perspective. The organisation had no interest in the process by which Claire's competency could be assured – it was merely concerned with the outcome.

Claire and I met to discuss and review the plan which required her to provide evidence that she had studied the mode and action of certain drugs, could successfully pass an assessment of her practical skills in drug administration and could present a written reflective account outlining where she had 'made the error'. I felt uncomfortable with this demand to 'confess' her error when the real value of reflective practice is as a tool to enhance learning.

To my surprise, and indeed pleasure, Claire took the 'confessional' reflective account that she had already written from her bag and tore it up. She had not felt comfortable writing it and now saw no value in it.

I journal:

> December 2003 – Claire and I met to look at her performance management plan. She was very positive in her outlook, had resolved and dealt with the experience and felt ready to move on. Her reflective account seems to suggest real learning from the experience. She surprised me when she said that in a way she was happy that the incident (drug error) had occurred as it made her think deeply and focus her practice. She said she now feels like a better nurse. We had quite a frank discussion about our relationship and Claire said that this episode has changed how she feels about me as her ward sister. She was unsure about me before, as she was very new to the ward. Now she feels able to come and talk to me and feels very supported on the ward. This pleases me a great deal! I asked Claire why she felt unsure of me before and I got the impression that she previously saw all 'managers' in that monitoring and surveillance role. Nursing still has a long way to go if it's ever to divorce itself from the old hierarchical notions of management control and agenda settings, not helped I'm sure by the recent introduction of the all-powerful and controlling 'Modern Matron' – what an oxymoron!

Claire's imposed performance management plan required that the organisation was given proof of the achievement of clear outcomes as a means of dealing with an area of Claire's practice that had caused concern. We achieved that. We had journeyed together towards a new understanding of the incident, and this enabled her to achieve real learning and a new, positive sense of self. Such commitment to the development of others is a crucial element in my own determination towards transformational leadership (Schuster 1994). Claire's learning was both on a practical level in terms of skill development (drug administration) but perhaps more importantly she had begun to develop the skills of self-reflection and analysis, useful in her wider daily life and practice. Claire is just one person in a large organisation not in tune with the concept of the learning organisation. Her learning may appear insignificant to some in the larger picture, but organisations can only learn through the individuals within it, and my desire, as a transformational leader, is to facilitate such learning (Senge 1990).

My experience with Claire taught me that I can resist the organisation's attempt to use me inappropriately to monitor and report on the practice of others. I felt liberated from fear that the organisation might view me negatively, or even punish me, mindful that such fear is endemic within nurses, characteristic of subordinate and oppressed people (Roberts 1983, 2000) fuelled by a culture of blame and shame.

Challenging the transactional

During the final months of my leadership programme, my attention turned towards my unsatisfactory relationship with Ann, the ward manager. A crisis was looming in our relationship. It had become increasingly challenging for me to perform as a transformational leader in an area where she was intensely transactional towards the staff. Ann's transactional nature was increasingly causing unrest among the staff, who disparagingly compared her transactional leadership style with my different approach. My journal entries had previously alluded to Ann's actions, but at the end of a week in February my journal contained an entry that proved to be the set of experiences that eventually led to my final determination to tackle the problem.

I journal:

> February 2004 – I have had a very unsettling week at work and think the time has come to do something about the problem with Ann (the ward manager). I again raised the problem of the reduction in the number of staff on the ward and how difficult it now is to manage the workload. 'Well it's matron's decision to save money,' she said. Surely we can do something about this, I thought, but she is adamant that matron has spoken so we just have to get on with it. Ann 'reprimanded' me this week for telling a consultant on Monday morning that, as I have just had a week off work, I did not yet know about his patient and his progress in the last week. Apparently, I should have pretended that I did know in order to keep him happy, and the fact that the consultant behaved in a boorish manner and stormed off the ward in full hearing of everyone doesn't seem to be a problem! I initially thought Ann had changed when I observed her telling Lisa (a staff nurse) that as the patient's named nurse she could make the decision herself as to whether a patient could have visitors out of hours. How wrong I was! When Lisa made the decision, Ann overruled her in the hearing of the visitor, other staff and patients, telling her she had made the 'wrong decision'! Lisa was very upset and said she felt totally humiliated. I know that these are just typical examples of the transactional management I work with and I don't think it can carry on like this. I don't see how we can work collaboratively when her approach is so different from mine. I'm feeling a bit adrift at the moment and I need some guidance through this particular swamp.

Avoidance of the problem was not an option. I spent the following week feeling very unsure of myself. I recognised that I was feeling continually oppressed by what I saw as Ann's higher status, despite the fact that she only worked part time on the ward. Ann had set the agenda for any meetings I had with her and so was prepared in advance. I usually had no prior knowledge of what was to be discussed, placing me at a disadvantage. I shared my frustration in the guided reflection group. I was enabled to see that in a sense I had *allowed* myself to be oppressed and that it was my own ineffectual action that had exacerbated the situation. By not acting, I had almost helped Ann to behave in her transactional manner to the detriment of myself and everyone else on the ward. Although I now felt confident to approach this challenge, it was at this point that the role of my reflective guide within the community of inquiry was crucial in challenging and supporting me to act. I absorbed the idea of 'front foot thinking'[2] – notably taking the initiative and being prepared rather than being caught on the back foot, reactive, defensive and uncertain. I recognised that while I had become a transformative leader for those I work with, I still felt restrained at a macro level, where oppression theory would explain my feelings of being controlled somewhat by Ann with her senior position to mine (Farrell 2001). The community's prompting gave me the courage to resist the perceived oppression, adopt front foot thinking and tackle my feelings of disempowerment head on.

I arranged a meeting with Ann to discuss the problems on the ward. Interestingly, when I asked, her immediate reaction was to ask if there was anything she should be worried about! This was always my previous reaction to her, so this turnaround signified to me a real difference in the power differential. The meeting proved a real insight into Ann's character and it confirmed for me how truly transactional she really was. Our conversation around the issue of a reduction in staff on the ward revealed that as a nurse she felt that it was unacceptable but felt powerless to do anything about it. Ann seemed to agree with me that the organisation appeared to be aiming for the cheapest and lowest standard of nursing care considered acceptable rather than reach the highest possible standard. She felt that she could do nothing about staffing reductions, even in her position as manager. Ann clearly displayed the feelings of oppression generated by those above her but wished to keep the issue at arm's length.

Topics of disagreement emerged. Her stance on my interaction with a consultant had not changed and she still felt I was wrong and should have been prepared 'to play the game' as she phrased it. This was complete anathema to me as I have long since rejected the historical unquestioned hierarchical relationship which underpinned the doctor–nurse relationship and strongly believe that nursing must shift from a position of traditional medical dominance and subordination (Stein 1967).

Finally, her reversal of Lisa's decision concerning the visitor was discussed, but Ann was adamant that she had to step in as Lisa had, in her opinion, made the wrong decision. In a truly telling comment, Ann stated that Lisa *was* empowered but only as much as she would allow her to be! I was keenly aware that managerial practices that criticise, punish and give little praise mitigate strongly against any feelings of empowerment among staff, and it seemed that this incident had been a clear portrayal of such restrictive practice. It is the provision of opportunities for nurses to participate more fully in decision-making and to develop a greater work ownership that denotes a move to a power relationship of shared responsibility (Lewis and Urmston 2000). This is my preferred transformational stance but it did not appear to be a stance shared by Ann. I attempted to encourage Ann to discuss our differing approaches to leadership as a means to begin the collaborative process. To my surprise, Ann began our conversation by demanding to know why I felt the need to 'rock the boat' as she phrased it. I must admit that I was quite pleased by her question. I had dared to be different and she had recognised that. She quickly followed this question by the recommendation that I needed to develop more people skills! She revealed she would prefer me to act in a transactional manner as she did.

It was patently evident to me that Ann symbolised the transactional organisation. She had no insight into her role as the preserver of the hierarchical structures and the status quo. She demonstrated no evidence of any empowerment in her role and seemed to have accepted this as the norm. Empowerment, while difficult to define, is more easily explained by its absence (Lewis and Urmston 2000). Ann exuded powerlessness, helplessness, hopelessness, alienation, victimisation, subordination, oppression, paternalism and marginalisation — all symbols of a lack of sense of control over one's life and role (Wallerstein and Bernstein 1988, Gibson 1991, Tones and Tilford 1994). By her actions, she was transferring these feelings of disempowerment to the staff below her but exhibited no recognition of this. I now recognised that this, too, has been my position prior to the course. Ann's higher status to my own would no longer constrain me. Her compliance with organisational objectives seemed a prison of her own making from which I was striving to escape. Tschudin (1999) suggests that many managers continue in their roles only because they remain muzzled and stay silent. It seems very obvious to me who actually applies the muzzle, but the unstinting consent of most managers to the process of muzzling now both saddens and horrifies me. At this point, I truly felt that the leadership programme had enabled me to fashion a valuable and increasingly impenetrable space between myself and the organisation where I no longer needed to remain silent to survive.

I knew that the different leadership approaches of Ann and myself needed to be resolved. Although, as a transformational leader, my preferred option would be to work collaboratively together, I recognised that this road would be fraught with difficulties. Honey (2002) notes that intransigent and dogmatic people like Ann are often very difficult to influence and are highly resistant to persuasion. I would need all of my negotiating and collaborative skills in the future months but I looked forward to the challenge as a new learning opportunity not only for myself but also for Ann. Although I remained a little apprehensive of what the future may bring, I felt determined to persist in what would probably be hard times – one of Schuster's (1994) leadership capacities. Ann and I agreed to meet weekly for briefing and discussion at a set time and this signified a positive move towards developing a collaborative relationship infused with leadership values. However, life is always unpredictable, and events were about to take an unexpected turn. Ann was absent from work for an extended period with a stress-related illness and then the final act in this particular chapter of experience took place.

Ringing the change

I journal:

> March 2004 – Ann rang me today to tell me that she has resigned from her job as ward manager. I don't feel a bit surprised though perhaps a little sad that I have been unable to guide her towards the transformational leadership trail. She didn't really tell me why she has resigned, but I wonder if she has finally realised that part-time transactionalism will never work on a ward where a transformational ward sister leads the staff. I think to be a transformational leader within the harsh transactional environment of the NHS requires real courage and determination and perhaps Ann is not ready or willing to take on the challenge. I think that's a real missed opportunity because, as a team, we could have been a very powerful combination in the organisation. It will be interesting to see if I am successful in my application for the ward manager's post. Maybe the organisation is not yet ready to accept me into the echelons of management. Will they think that I won't fit in with my different ideas and leadership style? Time will tell but whatever happens, I have already found and opened the greatest prize of all – being true at last to my own self and my desired practice and beliefs.

Perhaps my persistent pressure on Ann to embrace a transformational style contributed to her stress. But I am not taking responsibility for that. I know that transformational leadership cannot be compromised. My vision for my work practices is now clearly defined and I hold true passion for my leadership role (Schuster 1994). Had Ann and I succeeded in sharing the vision, I believe that it would have provided the focus and energy for mutual learning. Senge (1990) writes that a shared vision is the first step in allowing people who mistrusted each other to begin to work together since it creates a common identity. It was my concern for the people I work with, and not merely my own well-being, that led me to tackle the problem with Ann. This concern for the whole led me to reflect that my actions have moved significantly from being previously based on self-protection and promotion towards actions that now firmly embrace the needs of others. As a response to my deep concern for the ward staff, my transformational desire to help Ann to develop as an effective leader meant that I needed to act. I felt secure enough in my own desire and beliefs to tackle the problem and was prepared to see it through.

Learning the art of transformational leadership has shifted my locus of control from one that was external to strongly internal (Oberle 1991). This means that I no longer feel my actions are controlled by external events over which I have no control. I am no longer a passive recipient – rather I have become an active agent for change. This new stance, enhanced as it is by the concept of front foot thinking, means that my internal locus of control has made me much more self-directed and motivated and able to challenge and resist where necessary. My experience with Ann and the actions I took are perhaps, for me, the defining moment of my leadership journey so far, since they demonstrate perhaps the two most critical aspects of my now desired practice – the desire to be concerned for and to develop others, and the knowledge and confidence to challenge the (seemingly) all-powerful organisation when I believe it is morally necessary to do so. As Chambers (2002: 128) so pertinently remarked, 'The mark of a true leader is someone who sees the vision, shares it with others and takes them on a journey that makes it all happen.' The challenge for nursing has been set. Game on.

The continuing journey

I got the ward manager's position. I am increasingly confident to accept and welcome new problems and leadership challenges as learning opportunities rather than as threats to my role as previously. Such challenges and opportunities arise frequently and reflect deep tensions within the organisation (Bennis and Nanus 1985). My current leadership challenge relates to what is often the most problematic of all leadership concerns – the nature of human beings and their individual behavioural responses.

I journal:

> April 2004 – Just as I thought all was well, an old problem has reared its head again! I thought Moira was going to settle down after coming back from long-term sick leave. How wrong was I! – she's only been back a while and already she's upsetting everyone as she apparently did before with her comments and attitude. Just as I felt the team was really working well! She's upset the staff nurses and the HCAs [health care assistant] to the point where Sally was crying in the corridor about her, and the atmosphere on the ward is extremely tense. I need to think how to tackle this and consider why it is happening. What can I do to resolve this? Perhaps Moira feels really unhappy at work or uncertain about her role. Perhaps she needs a new challenge. Maybe it's not her fault as such. We need to talk and see if we can resolve this once and for all. I see Moira as a valuable member of the ward team – she works hard and the patients all like her. I want her to feel supported and welcomed by the other staff but it seems she doesn't at the moment. Does she feel undervalued? Is she frustrated as a HCA? I'll talk to her when I go back to work and see if we can work this out together.

How do I respond to Moira as a transformational leader? It may well be that Moira is cantankerous, over-controlling and unable to grasp the concept of team working. However, rather than ascribe all the blame to her, as I perhaps previously would have, I am now considering my own contribution to the problem – am I doing something wrong? What is my part in this as a leader? Simply blaming Moira seems merely an avoidant option at the moment. This issue, while not resolved as yet, reminds me that knowing myself as a leader remains precarious in the face of emotional reaction. The difference is that I now see the tensions even if I still struggle at times to respond congruently with my leadership values. Peck (1978) writes that once we accept and understand that life is difficult, then paradoxically life is no longer difficult. However, I wonder if the NHS is truly ready for genuine leaders who challenge the transactional nature of the health service? The answer to this is probably 'not yet' but I am optimistic it will come. I feel rather like a missionary in the field in my own workplace, filled with a zeal sending out ripples to infect and eventually shift the transactional world.

Conclusion

Martha engages with her vision of becoming a *transformational* leader inspired by Schuster's interpretation of what that means. She comes to reflexively recognise herself as changed, different from her transactional colleagues who typify the organisation. She is of service to her junior staff, mindful of the undercurrents and tensions that have previously separated her from them. The word 'trust' looms large and underpins the development of relationship.

At first Martha's staff did not trust her because they had come to view management with suspicion. Slowly she built trust and with it the possibility of creating a learning organisation. When people are beaten down you cannot expect them to be committed. They have sunk into resignation, compliance and worse, apathy. Investment cannot be rushed. Leaders need to be present on the shop floor where it matters, so they know the smell of the place, so they can understand, so they are visible, so they can demonstrate credibility, so they can support and care and so they can create a learning community with every action they take.

The journey of becoming is a narrative. Indeed practice becomes a narrative continually unfolding once we have learnt to pay attention and reflect on its significance. As Martha says, 'I see the tensions', illuminating her becoming aware of herself as a leader within practice. It reflects how leadership is only possible when one is mindful of self as a leader. She inculcates her values of leadership until she becomes it as if it is natural. She cannot become complacent because as she says 'even if I still struggle at times to respond congruently with my leadership values'. As it is, her leadership is inchoate.

Reflection

- What insights do you draw from Martha's narrative?
- Consider Schuster's attributes – are they easy to understand and apply to your own leadership?
- To what extent do you recognise the transactional organisation?

Notes

1. Numerous definitions of clinical supervision exist, with the elements of professional learning and support, development of knowledge and competence, a means of encouraging self-assessment and the use of analytical and reflective skills being particularly evident (NHSME (National Health Service Management Executive) 1993).
2. See page 56.

3 The Learning Organisation

In her narrative (Chapter 2), Martha sought to establish the learning organisation (LO) within her practice. Senge (1990: 3) defined a LO as 'one where people continually expand their capacities to create the results they truly desire, where new and expansive patterns of thinking are nurtured, where collective aspiration is set free, and where people are continually learning how to learn together'. It offers the leader both a visionary and operational template to fulfil their leadership role.

The five disciplines

Senge identified five interlinking disciplines that constitute the LO: vision, mental models, systems thinking, team learning and personal mastery. However, I consider leadership to be a sixth discipline, one that facilitates the whole (Figure 3.1). Each discipline is fluid, shifting in response to the environment, and in dynamic relationship with the other disciplines. As such, they cannot be seen as separate but as a dynamic whole.

Vision

> Believe in the vision of you
> Practice the vision
> Become the vision
>
> *Jones and Jones (1996: 47)*

Vision is the foundation stone for the LO. Senge (1990: 9) writes, 'When there is a genuine vision, people excel and learn, not because they are told to, but because they want to.' Constructing a genuine vision builds commitment because everybody associated with practice is involved. Visions are inspirational. Constructing a vision brings people together in collective

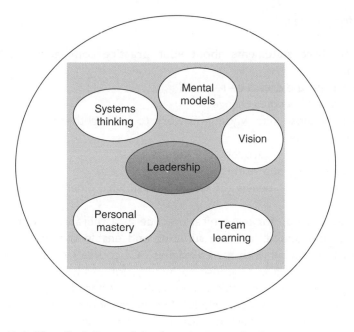

Figure 3.1 The disciplines of the learning organisation

enterprise towards a shared vision to guide practice. Visions create possibilities, excite the imagination and constantly challenge people to move beyond their current thinking and practices. By holding a vision, the values reflected within it are more likely to be realised simply because people know what they are trying to achieve. Vision is both intellectual and heartfelt. Visions reflect and nurture integrity. Visions focus and liberate personal responsibility. When people can act in ways concordant with their values then internal conflict is reduced. The world becomes a better place. A vision must also be a reflection of current reality so that people can relate to it, rather than being a beautiful fantasy clearly beyond the realms of practice. Yet as Greenleaf writes (2002: 30), 'not much happens without a dream'.

Martin Luther King Jr[1] said, 'I have a dream that my four little children will one day live in a nation where they will not be judged by the color of their skin, but by the content of their character. I have a dream that one day every valley shall be exalted, every hill and mountain shall be made low, the rough places will be made straight and the glory of the Lord shall be revealed and all flesh shall see it together. I have a dream that one day on the red hills of Georgia, the sons of former slaves and the sons of former slave owners will be able to sit together at the table of brotherhood.'

Try it for yourself:

- Write three statements about your practice commencing 'I have a dream'.
- How might the dream be realised?
- What would need to change?
- Then ask those with whom you work to get together and do this as a group exercise.
- Share and dialogue around your results.
- Then write a group vision.
- After one month review the vision and ask what difference it has made.

My personal vision for my clinical practice as a therapist and as a nurse can be simply stated: 'to ease suffering and enable the other to grow, in mutual endeavour with my colleagues'. Of course I could expand this vision, adding detail in response to inquiry, for example, 'What do you mean by words such as suffering and healing?' It begs the question, 'How much detail should a vision include?' My glib response would be no more than a sheet of A4 because it must have impact and be read in a glance rather than turn over pages. What makes a vision valid? I know my vision resonates with the WHO (World Health Organisation) vision of palliative care in particular with its focus on easing suffering. Holding a personal vision I have a deep sense of purpose as I approach each clinical encounter. As such I am more mindful and more likely to live the vision. I am also better able to contribute to any team or organisational vision.

Marina felt she once had a vision but it had withered within the transactional culture. She wrote a poem:

> Day one the tutor asked
> what is your vision?
> and I felt an awkward itch
> deep down inside
> I tried to let it pass but it persisted and hurt.
>
> I had a vision once, you see
> clear bright, so well defined
> but somehow it got mangled
> wilted, withered, nearly died
> once my life force, now my pain.
>
> It was so beautiful a vision!
> honoured women ... honoured life.

how did it get so crushed?
I'd nurtured it so long
and now I was in tatters.

In desperation to survive
I silenced it away
and all my vision stood for
somehow, sadly went astray.

Vision opens a gate to meaning. Meaning is the powerful attractor around which inherent order is patterned (Wheatley 1999). As a leader of a community hospital I asked the staff, 'Tell me about your hospital vision.' In response I heard vague references to the Loeb Centre in New York and the idea of 'nursing as therapy'. The Loeb Centre was a nursing unit established in New York (Hall 1964, Alfano 1971) that was revolutionary in promoting nursing as a primary therapy. This vision had been adopted for the community hospital (Pearson 1983). The staff's vague responses suggested that imported visions grounded in lofty ideas perish when the soil is not adequately prepared or maintained. In response I again went about creating a collaborative vision for clinical practice. Large sheets of paper were pinned to the wall inviting staff to state their values about nursing practice at the hospital. Slowly people emerged from the woodwork to write. A buzz about the place. Stirrings of curiosity – 'what is our practice about?' The sheets were pinned to the wall for three months until full. Against this background of inquiry I felt the pulse of the place. I asked people to tell me their stories, prodding, what gives, what makes people tick. I feel its resistance, an intangible sense of having been through this once before and not again, of the wasted effort as the culture of 'holistic' nursing slipped back into a normality that was once both disappointing and a relief – the slide-back into what Grant and Greene (2001) term the average level of mediocrity (ALOM). Everything changes all the time. To remain static is to wither and die. Visions paint a bigger picture encouraging a more expansive view of self and practice. Visions are confrontational, confronting the practitioner who is happy curled up in the comfort of normal routine.

I wrote out the statements from the flipchart paper to circulate to all staff. We met and explored the statements. Heated debate followed – those for and against nursing development stood up. So much resistance surprised me but I was not daunted. I drafted a composite statement of our philosophy for practice or vision.[2] Through a series of team meetings we debated until consensus was realised. The vision was written in jargon-free language![3] In this way it cannot be resisted as someone else's vision. It forces ownership even on those practitioners who merely complied with the process. Now began the hard graft of realising the vision as a lived reality.

Consider the following:

- Where is the vision for your practice? Is it visible?
- When was it written?
- Who wrote it?
- Does it reflect your beliefs and values about practice?
- Does it say something about the aims and processes of practice?
- Does it say anything about roles and relationships between colleagues?
- Does it say anything about change and quality?
- Does it pay attention to wider organisational and societal expectations?

Vision leads to a deeper sense of vision than just clinical practice; it reaches the heart of being human. What does it mean to be a nurse, doctor or leader? The focus of values is on being, not doing. It is essentially an onto-logical quest, not an epistemological one. Our actions and behaviour stem from our values and beliefs. And yet we must always hold these values open for scrutiny, not as a dogma that leads to prejudice, intolerance and conflict. Yet it is not easy; it takes discipline, hard work and time.

Janet writes: Fritz (1989) explains leadership as this energy is what the vision does, rather than what the vision is. He talks of vision as a power, enabling one to reach through the ordinary to the extraordinary; the inner eye of vision able to conceive something clearly that does not yet exist, the energy for change and creativity. In the words of Wheatley (1999: 55), a vision 'should create a power, not a place, an influence, not a destination'.

Mental models

Mental models are the norms, values and assumptions that govern the way leaders see and respond to the world. However mental models are not easily shifted because they reflect who we are, especially when ways of being and doing in practice are deeply embodied and reinforced through normal patterns of relating. Through reflection, practitioners access and scrutinise their mental models for their congruency with desired leadership. Mental models can be accessed through the model for structured reflection cues:

- What factors influence the way I was/am feeling, thinking and responding to this situation?

- What are my underlying assumptions that govern my practice and what is the basis for these assumptions? How do I need to shift them in order to realise my leadership?[4]

List five assumptions that govern your practice. What is the basis for these assumptions? Are these assumptions appropriate for practice? Step back and take a good hard look at yourself. For example, one assumption might be that 'it's common sense to organise an organisation through hierarchy so there is a clear chain of command otherwise chaos would ensue'. A more transformational assumption might read, 'it's common sense to flatten the hierarchy and enable everybody to take responsibility for their own actions. In this way the best in people would surface'. Ask yourself, 'What actions would you as a leader take to support either of these assumptions? If you agree with it, how could you act to move from the first to the second assumption?' Thinking differently is the precursor for acting differently.

> Maya writes: My history of fear of getting things wrong, being rebuffed, being rejected and being seen as a freak has tended to keep me on safe predictable land or even retreat away from what I believe in to avoid pain. My mental models have historically impeded my growth.

Systems thinking

Whilst mental models focus practitioners to look inside themselves, systems thinking focuses practitioners to reveal and critique the background pattern of systems that organise practice. Systems are constructed to support the delivery of services. As Greenleaf writes (2002: 29), a leader needs to be more than inspirational. He needs structures. Undoubtedly, systems within large health care organisations are complex. They can be likened to machines made up of many parts. The transformational leader views systems as a whole and understands the relationship between different parts in contrast with a more mechanical perspective of focusing on specific parts that are disrupting the smooth running of the organisation. The problem with systems is that they can enforce conformity on people, reducing them to objects within the machine rather than humans. From this logic, humans are prone to error and mess up the system rather than the system being at fault. Clearly systems are essential in organising practice and yet systems need to be seen for what they are – supporting practice. Leaders are liberated from machine-like thinking to see the whole picture and the pattern within it. Systems tend to be rigid and unyielding. By loosening systems, everything becomes more flexible. This requires double feedback loops that not only monitor what is going on but constantly monitor the system itself for its appropriateness to monitor what it needs to monitor. This shifts a system from being static and self-confirming to being dynamic and adaptable.

Wheatley and Kellner-Rogers (1996: 41) write, 'stability is found in freedom, not in compliance or conformity. We may have thought that our organisation's survival was guaranteed by finding the right form and insisting that everyone fits into it. But sameness is not stability. It is individual freedom that creates stable systems. It is differentness that enables us to thrive.'

In liberating people and systems the organisation becomes more flexible and can embrace uncertainty and complexity confidently. It becomes more self-organising, letting go and flowing with uncertainty. As chaos theory teaches us, order patterns itself around meaning (Wheatley 1999). Senge (1990) viewed systems thinking as the fifth discipline, the one that holds the others together. The risk with systems is that they become ends in themselves, demanding conformity even when the system obstructs effective practice. To reiterate, perhaps it is easier to blame the human performance rather than the system even when it is known that most problems of performance are caused by the system. Through reflection systems can be understood and scrutinised for their value to facilitate the most effective practice. Leaders become political towards involvement in shifting systems as necessary.

Team learning

Vision, personal mastery, mental models and systems thinking all come into synergistic play through team learning. Team learning is how people learn together within a community of inquiry – the collaborative effort to realise shared vision. Senge (1990: 236) writes, 'Team learning is the process of aligning and developing the capacity of a team to create the results its members truly desire.' This becomes possible because such groups work through dialogue, reflection and deep trust. As such the mindful leader always seeks to create and sustain a learning community to enable others to reflect and to become mindful leaders.

Dialogue

Team learning is through dialogue. Dialogue is a particular way of conversing with self, others or text. Bohm (1996) notes that the word *dialogue* comes from the Greek *Dia-logus* – meaning flowing through – a stream of meaning flowing among and through us and between us. It is this flow that holds and directs the community of inquiry. Dialogue is also the talk that leaders use with everybody whether within a community of inquiry, in conversations with colleagues or patients, or at management meetings even when resisted by other more transactional types of talk.

Dialogue has a number of qualities (Bohm 1996):

- Commitment to work with others towards a consensus for a better world.
- Being aware of and suspending one's assumptions and prejudices (mental models) and being open to possibility.
- Proprioception of thinking – knowing where one's thinking is at any moment.
- Viewing experience as a learning opportunity free from attachment to ideas. Only then are people open to the possibilities within the moment and able to liberate self from habitual patterns of perceiving and responding to situations.
- Listening to each other with respect and engagement. Listening is empathic. It is enabling the other person to tell their story and connect with their experience. It is being open to what the other person is saying: suspending one's own agenda and self-concerns to hear clearly what the other is saying, sensing the underlying feelings, things that are not being said, picking up cues and reading signs.
- Having a mutual appreciation of dialogue and its *rules* and taking both individual and collective responsibility for ensuring its integrity.

Working with others towards consensus is the essence of community. Everyone has a voice to be respected. Dialogue encourages voice to be expressed and valued. The process of dialogue enables our assumptions to be 'lifted' and scrutinised for their appropriateness without attachment. Proprioception is itself mindfulness, an intuitive sense of knowing where your mind is at any given moment. Dialogue is always creative. As Tufnell and Crickmay (2004: 41) observe, 'creating becomes a conversation when we enter a dialogue with whatever we are doing. In this conversing we are drawn along in the moment by moment flow of sensation, interchange and choice, rather than following a predetermined intention or idea. Conversations grow as we listen and explore – a constantly shifting process of discovery that changes in momentum, rhythm, clarity or chaos as we work.'

Within a transactional world dominated by patterns of communication concerned with self-interest and control, dialogue is rare, perhaps not surprisingly given its subtlety. Go to any management meeting and simply listen to the pattern of talk. Some people are quiet and others talk every opportunity to voice their opinion. People compete to talk, to get their point across, without listening to what has been said before, even interrupting before the other has finished. Few people are open to possibility due to a preoccupation with their own agenda. Dialogue is expansive, pulling open the big picture whereas other forms of talk tend to focus on the small picture.

Within the learning community people relate to each other in ways that facilitate openness, curiosity and reflection. As Wheatley and Kellner-Rogers write (1996: 100), 'If we take time to reflect together on who we are and who we would choose to become, we will be led into the territory where change originates.' In this sense dialogue is a collective reflection on reflection, drawing out insights that enable growth of the people involved. Within the learning community, its members ask pertinent questions, shape new patterns, shift tradition, bend authority, surface assumptions and unlearn ingrained responses. Everyone contracts to support each other. Wheatley writes (1999: 130), 'we have to help one another notice when we fall back into old behaviours. We will all slip back into the past – that is unavoidable – but when this happens, we agree to counsel one another with a generous spirit.'

In this way, practice is always changing, growing and chipping away at old defunct patterns that cling on through inertia to change. Around the table everyone is connected within the whole. Gilley (1997: 49) writes, 'As we seek connection rather than separation, differences are honoured as part of our uniqueness that is the spirit of each of us. We create connection when we let go of attachment to a particular way of doing things and focus instead on achieving our purpose.'

Of course people may have an attachment to a particular view, but these are lifted into perspective and held loosely. Any conflict of view is simply surfaced as a difference that we work together to find the best solution for. Such dialogue becomes normal in everyday conversations. 'We grow, by the gaze of one another' (Cixous 1999: 7).

> Lynda writes: I chaired the meeting completely differently from before, encouraging people to listen with engagement and respect. One person came up to me afterwards and thanked me for the meeting, the most constructive meeting she had attended. She had felt engaged and motivated. I did as well. I couldn't believe how different the meeting could be and with such positive outcomes.

Positive feedback

An aspect of team learning is feedback. I ask aspiring leaders to brainstorm the impact of receiving either positive or negative feedback about their performance:

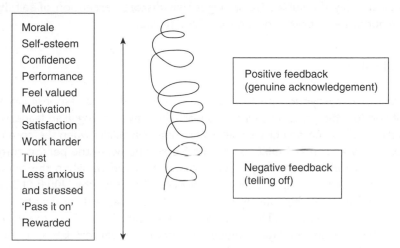

Morale
Self-esteem
Confidence
Performance
Feel valued
Motivation
Satisfaction
Work harder
Trust
Less anxious
and stressed
'Pass it on'
Rewarded

Positive feedback
(genuine acknowledgement)

Negative feedback
(telling off)

Reviewing the list, the leaders are stunned about the apparent impact of positive or negative feedback on their performance. I use the example of a smile and frown – the impact of that on self and that something so apparently simple is so profound in influencing self and performance.

I am mindful of ideas such as the butterfly effect. Wikipedia notes: 'The butterfly effect is a phrase which encapsulates the more technical notion of sensitive dependence on initial conditions in chaos theory. Small variations of the initial condition of a nonlinear dynamical system may produce large variations in the long term behaviour of the system.'[5]

Hence, a smile and eye contact rather than eye avoidance or a frown will radically shift the conditions of practice within a positive amplifying spiral across the organisation. Being smiled at the person is more likely to smile to others – 'to pass it on' creating a positive shock wave through the organisation. Leaders like positive feedback yet are tough when necessary, tough on issues soft on people. People who feel valued are less anxious releasing energy for enhanced performance.

Personal mastery

Personal mastery is the art of holding creative tension – the tension between a vision and an understanding of current reality. In other words the focus for reflection as people seek to realise their vision as a lived reality. Senge (1990: 7) notes, 'The discipline of personal mastery is continually clarifying and deepening our personal vision, of focusing our energies, of developing patience and of seeing reality objectively'. Holding creative tension is being mindful of self within the moment. The idea of seeing reality objectively is to clear away the subjective smudges that distort perception of self. It is also about being poised or emotionally intelligent.

Leadership

In principle, everyone within the LO is a leader and takes responsibility for self and for the group as a whole to learn. However, recognised leadership guidance of the community enhances learning, especially when the community is newly formed. Reflection can be frustrating when the person comes to understand herself and yet sees no way forward or when the person berates herself through the reflective process. Loori writes (2004: 118), 'As the creative leadership journey evolves, the leaders stumble against barriers that hinder the journey. These barriers are woven deep within them, triggered by patterns of relating embedded within the everyday fabric of transactional organisational life. But what happens when you are not aware of the barrier in the first place? How can you deal with it? This is where creative feedback is invaluable. It can show you your sticking places and blind spots. It's hard to go through this process alone, without a teacher or someone to provide insight into your art. That's like the eye trying to see itself'.

> Karen writes: Guidance helps me to surface the limitations that I put on myself. The group is small. There is a real sense that we all learn from each other's experiences. There is a willingness to share our thoughts. I feel safe exposing my thoughts to them, liberating my energy entangled in anxiety and seeing a way forward.

Besides the obvious benefit of being within a group of like-minded people experiencing similar journeys, guidance is necessary to enhance learning through reflection for a number of reasons:

- to challenge and support the aspiring leaders
- to work through emotional tension in order to hold creative tension
- to reflect on deeper, more critical levels to reveal how becoming a leader is constrained by embodiment, force and tradition
- to co-create meaning with one's peers and guides whereby individual horizons are transcended in common purpose

- to find one's own way (when it is seems easier to be told)
- to take courage and persevere when the going is hard against the apparently unyielding wall of reality
- to re-moralise a self that has become demoralised through working in oppressive (transactional) systems (Frank 2002)

Guidance is disturbing people, ruffling the smooth surface, and *nudging* them into new ways of seeing. Guides help leaders find their own creative path through the dense transactional undergrowth.

Rowena writes: Deeper insights and more critical levels of inquiry can be achieved with the assistance of a 'guide' to channel and encourage the reflective process. Without guidance, self-reflection can be limited by feelings of unease and remorse arising from the self-scrutiny involved. As Johns (2004a: 37) observes, 'the deeper we go, the more defended we are likely to be'. The combination of objectivity, critical analysis and attentive listening has become addictive. In terms of developing my leadership practice I increasingly recognise it is an indulgence I can ill-afford to do without.

Guides are particularly mindful to walk the talk and lead as a leader. Guides share their own narratives, putting themselves out there, being vulnerable and transparent.

Wheatley (1999: 130) informs, 'In organisations where leaders do not practice what they preach, there are terrible disabling consequences ... they have got to really, genuinely, walk the talk, practice what they preach, live out what they say ... in a chaotic world, we need leaders. But we don't want bosses. We need leaders to help us develop the clear identity that lights the dark moments of confusion. We need leaders to support us as we learn how to live by our values.'

Guides walk alongside the community members/aspiring leaders, challenging and supporting them along the way, helping them understand, expanding their perspectives, holding their anxiety, infusing them with courage as their shoulders sag, helping them to shift the boulders that appear to block the path, supporting them when they are knocked down and cheering their success. Aspiring leaders would quickly sense any contradiction in the guide's behaviour! No room for complacency, and yet contradictions are good learning moments.

The development of leadership is not the guide's responsibility. He is simply of service to guide each emerging leader individually and collectively to realise their leadership vision. Not *his* vision, although clearly it is imperative his own vision is aligned with that of the emerging leaders.

The guide's role is *to hold the learning space* and create the conditions within the learning environment whereby the aspiration to become a leader becomes possible. Creating the community cannot merely be a nice idea; it has to be actively constructed. However, this may not be easy as it goes against the grain of mainstream university education, just as it does within the transactional health care organisation.

The demand on the guide to tell them *what to do* or *how to be* can be considerable especially when team learning is new and people haven't learnt to dialogue or take responsibility for self-performance within the community. Perhaps then, a more didactic approach can be appropriate, providing the leader is mindful of the risk of imposing her own perceptions on others – of shaping the path they should take.

Marie writes: Our guide outlined the idea of reflective practice as a way of focusing and appreciating this tension, and as a way to begin to 'test' ourselves as leaders within everyday practice. Through reflection we can begin to give form and meaning to our visions of leadership in dialogue with the vast literature that lay daunting on my study desk at home. Why can't he just tell us what leadership is?

He doesn't tell because it would contradict what leadership seeks to enable. Leadership is thus concerned with creating and sustaining a learning environment based on mutual responsibility to support each other and shared success. Shared success legitimises that individuals within the organisation have their own criteria for aspiration and that such criteria should be acknowledged and valued by the organisation whilst expecting the individual to work towards organisational aspiration.

Mick Cope gives this idea substance with the 3 Vs (Cope 2001):

- The extent to which you share the same values and beliefs as the others in the relationship.
- The extent to which care and consideration are demonstrated with the result that people feel valued.
- The extent to which you demonstrate that you understand the value the other person adds to the relationship.

This model captures three crucial elements of leadership – vision, investment in others and support. Cope (2001: 185) describes shared success as balancing high advocacy with high inquiry:

- Advocacy: making sure other people know what you want and need by having the courage to tell them.
- Inquiry: understanding other people's goals, dreams and desires by showing them consideration and seeking to understand what success means for them.

Conclusion

The LO offers a compelling vision for leaders to create and sustain a learning environment where people can grow and establish the collaborative community. Indeed creating and sustaining the LO becomes the primary task of leadership simply because within it leadership can itself flourish. This is actualised through leadership, personal mastery and team learning. In this process, vision, mental models and systems are aligned towards realising the vision as a lived reality. Creating and sustaining the LO itself becomes part of the vision.

It makes utter sense to enable leadership development through the LO. Then leaders can rehearse creating it in practice (see Appendix A1).

Reflection

- Consider how you might establish a potent LO in your own practice.
- Observe patterns of 'talk' at meetings you are involved with. Imagine how different the meeting would be through dialogue.
- If you are leading a meeting, introduce and use dialogue. Reflect on its impact.

Notes

1. www.brainyquotes.com
2. At that time I used the expression 'philosophy for practice'. I now prefer 'vision statement'.
3. The vision is published in *Becoming a reflective practitioner* (2nd edition) (Johns 2004a) together with an analysis of what constitutes a valid vision.
4. See Appendix 1 figure.
5. http://en.wikipedia.org/wiki/Butterfly_effect

4 It's Automatic, Isn't It?

Introduction

The different theories about the nature of leadership can confuse the aspiring leader. Which to choose? Each is compelling in its own way. Alison was inspired by the idea of servant leader. As you read, consider the way the attributes of servant leadership are threaded through the narrative:

Attributes of servant leadership

- The servant leader is servant-first, committed to enabling others' growth needs to be met before her own. Yet in ensuring others needs, the servant leader's needs are also met. As people grow they also become servant leaders.
- The servant leader shows others the way; this showing gives them their 'lead'. They can show the way because of their vision and foresight that marks them out to 'lead'.
- The servant leaders listen first because they are mindful, compassionate and wise. They can listen because that is their agenda. They are not driven by ego concerns.
- The servant leader puts herself forward. She is destined to lead. She has the courage, poise and resilience to take the risk even when the future is uncertain and yet she has a better-than-average grasp of the unforeseeable. It is an intuitive refinement of consciousness gained through listening, empathy and acceptance of how things are. She has an intuitive feel for patterns and does not suffer delusion.
- The servant leader knows how to prioritise and persuade people. Because of her openness, honesty, consistency, vulnerability and presence people trust her to lead them, even when leadership is subtle. Leadership is truly spiritual.
- The servant leader is grounded in loving and caring communities. This is the basic ground that nourishes and sustains such leadership and shapes servant institutions.

> Alison writes: Sitting in a drab classroom, I wait for the programme director to arrive. I feel nervous and excited at the same time. I am a ward manager employed by a primary care trust (PCT). The ward is an assessment and treatment unit for people aged sixty-five and above with organic and functional illness. I have worked for the trust for ten years since qualifying as a registered mental health nurse. I manage a team of twenty nursing staff, qualified and unqualified. I use the ward manager to reflect what I was doing prior to the leadership course. I am also a leader. It's automatic, isn't it?

An emphasis on leadership can be traced back to the Department of Health (1999) statement: *Ward managers have a pivotal role in national health organisations and therefore a key focus for developing leadership.* Professional carers, whether they like it or not, are required to demonstrate leadership qualities since others will expect guidance, advice, enthusiasm, belief, confirmation and support, and the lack of a formal leadership title does not absolve one from leadership responsibilities. More importantly is the ability of nurses' leaders to have a direct impact on the standard of patient care (Cook 2001). The government has purported to understand and recognise the unique role of the ward sister in the provision of leadership at ward level, describing it as critical to the quality of patient care, treatment and outcomes to staff morale and the learning climate. The government further acknowledged that ward sisters are undervalued and do not get the recognition they deserve despite being the backbone of the NHS and the hub of the wider clinical team. Leadership then is undoubtedly required of me but living out the role seems fraught with potential difficulties.

This responsibility to be a leader knocks on my professional door. It concerns me because I was promoted in a short space of time and enlisted onto a first-line management course without drawing breath. Looking back, it felt as though I was caught up in a whirlwind, indoctrinated into management before I had chance to find out who I was. It was not my ambition to become a ward manager; I was quite happy being a charge nurse. The opportunity arose and I took it. At times I feel as if I have compromised my values. I came into nursing because I love it. I love caring and being with people. Now as a ward manager I have less contact as I have so much managerial stuff to do and I miss working with patients. It would be easy to be resentful of my position but I strive to retain the passion. Perhaps leadership is the way?

Now, as I write, I am mindful of being a leader or perhaps of becoming a leader inspired by the idea of servant leadership. As I read Greenleaf

(2002), I strove to make sense or find meaning in these ideas for they were not easy to grasp, notably the idea of service in an organisational culture that is completely driven from the top down. Yet *being of service* feels right. I touch its ideological edge and feel an opening of possibility within me. My reading of servant leadership convinces me that I want to lead like that.

Normal strife

When I walk onto the ward in the morning I am mindful of creating and sustaining a collaborative community. I take my cues from the smiles and greetings or not, as the case may be. It hasn't always been like that. This was one of *those* days. By the look on a colleague's face I sense that something's wrong. I am intuitive like that. Sure enough, when time allowed, Mary, a nursing auxiliary, came to see me, banging the door shut, dropping herself into a chair, none too delicately. 'I'm bloody fed up with this place. I'm thinking of leaving.' Mary always starts with this kind of sentence when something has upset her. I'm thinking, *Oh God, now what*, although I do not say this. Mary launches into a tirade of accusations. I let her vent her anger, trying to get to the crux of the matter. It transpires that she felt her care of a patient was being thwarted by, in her opinion, less knowledgeable nurses. Mary's area of interest lies in wound care. She is very competent and has attended relevant courses and infection control meetings. She had drawn up a care plan for a patient's leg wound but believes that a particular staff nurse has deliberately ignored it. The staff nurse in question also has an interest in wound care. Mary believes her knowledge is superior and that the staff nurse is using the wrong dressings.

My irritation rises. This is not a problem I have time for. Yet I feel angry that Mary's care of the patient is being compromised. I need to fix it quickly so the ward can run smoothly. I suggest we talk to the staff nurse concerned. Mary does not want to confront her, stating, 'I have to work with her and you're not always around.' That sentence should have alerted me but I gave it no thought. It was not to be until months later, when I revisited this sentence, that I saw it more mindfully.

At the time I needed to appease Mary. My need to fix it was strong and the pressure on my time influenced my actions. Together we agreed to contact the wound care specialist nurse to assist us in drawing up a care plan. I put my name on it so that others were unlikely to challenge it, and indeed they did not. It gave authority to our plan, silencing doubting voices. That is how authority works with its sharp edge of coercion. I had no time for persuasion.

Sharing the experience in group reflection, I felt ashamed of my abuse of my position and power concerning the care plan. The consequences taught

Mary little, other than I would collude with her and manipulate other staff. This is not the way of the servant leader. I need to foster community, not manipulation. But then I was not leading; I was managing in a transactional manner. Did I consider the effect on other staff? No. I recognised that my need for control had a direct result of acting insensitively towards colleagues. Now I can see it. Before I hadn't. Reflection had opened my eyes as uncomfortable as that felt. The issue is, can I let go of my need to command in order to use my power to enable others to grow?

I thought I was being sensitive to Mary's request not to challenge the staff nurse in trying to understand her predicament. However, if I am honest, it was easier to agree to her request than face a confrontation. So why did I avoid it? Habit, I guess. Other nurses, including myself, tend to avoid situations that are likely to result in disharmony. Yet I can see that avoidance is a perverse caring. I can identify with Valentine (1994) when she expressed that nurses are supposed to be caring and that conflict is often perceived as non-caring. She wrote that twenty years ago and yet it seems nothing has changed. If anything it has got worse as the transactional culture gets even more transactional in its anxiety over targets and resources.

Yet conflict must be expected in a dynamic organisational environment and can be a motivator for change and growth. From a leadership perspective conflict points out what needs to be addressed and should be approached from a positive stance (Johns 2013). Perhaps then, at the start of my journey, I was not ready to change. I certainly was not skilled in managing conflict.

I recognised the significance of referent power[1] in my relationship with staff to persuade or influence rather than to command and control them. I saw the value of community to establish collaborative ways of working based on mutual responsibility and thick trust towards shared success. Cope (2001) describes trust as central to productive relationships and sharing goals. Mary has historically proved to be trustworthy. I had no reason not to trust the staff nurse; she is known for acting in the patient's best interest. However, she tends to see things in black and white and refuses to discuss grey areas. At that time the critical parent within me could quite happily have throttled her. But as Crowe (1999) suggests, strangling isn't an option. With hindsight, the patient may have benefited from a team approach to wound care.

I wrote in my journal that day:

> I get so fed up of staff tittle, tattling on each other. I wish I could shout, 'Will you all grow up!'

I imagine my guide in the leadership community saying 'Perhaps I need to let them.'

I sense how I am the critical parent, anxious, berating my aberrant children. I would like to be an adult, but being honest, I am not. The staff see me as a parent, and in turn they act as children in keeping with the paternalistic nature of the transactional organisation (Barker and Young 1994). With increasing awareness, I realise I am falling into a paternalistic trap of assuming my staff need direction to feel safe and to manage their anxieties (Holyoake 2000). I feel as if I'm a failure. Johns (2004a: 142) writes, 'The mindful practitioner chooses parent/child ego state to communicate as a matter of clinical judgement rather than as a reaction to anxiety.' I do not need to be a victim of the transactional work culture. I do have choice. I *can* learn to stand back, listen and see things for what they are and make choices rather than react and perpetuate the paternalistic status quo that is unsatisfactory for everybody. I sense creative tension scratching at my surface, like wearing a horsehair sweater over my naked skin. Whilst it irritates it also reminds me to pay attention. I must be patient with myself. The transactional world is deeply embodied within me. Argyris (1982) points out that the habitual ways of interacting are defensive routines to protect us from conflict, but alas, also prevent us from learning. I pull at these defensive routines, loosening them.

My pockets are full of pebbles that weigh me down. My leadership guide says, '*Show me.*' He turns them over and throws them into the pond. We watch the ripples spread out and rebound against the edge. Suddenly I feel lighter. He is the servant leader showing me the way when I had expected him to be judgemental and parental with me or telling me what to do to fix the situation. He just listened (just listened?), guiding me to explore how I might respond more congruently with my servant leader values. I sense his intuitive feel for Greenleaf's patterns, wisdom and compassion.

Yielding

A few months later. We are shortstaffed with only one qualified staff member on duty. It is ward round day, which takes most of the morning. The qualified nurse is removed from the clinical area during this time and I normally cover the ward. I am expecting an admission. I need to find staff for the night shift to cover sickness, and we are being visited by the Mental Health Act Commissioners. The new computers arrive and I get a splinter in my finger from rearranging the desks. The phone rings continuously. Families arrive for the ward round. The dietician requests a handover and the daily diary has mountains of requests to sort out. One of those days when you think, 'Please, God, don't let me forget anything.'

Management is a juggling act. How many plates can I juggle without dropping and breaking one?

In my journal I write:

> Someone brought me tea, thank you, wonderful person.

A simple thing but one I appreciated. Caring manifests itself in such small acts of service.

In the midst of this I receive a phone call from my manager, commanding me to go to the general ward to assess a patient and decide whether the patient would be suitable for admission to our ward. I explain the situation on the ward and say it would have to be later on in the day. I get the distinct feeling she isn't happy about this and tells me to go as soon as possible. I feel a prickle of resentment, thinking why can't she bloody well do it, instead of sitting in her office giving out orders if it's *that* urgent! I didn't say that to her. I buttoned the emotion. I know *actions have consequences*. My childish temper tantrum is quelled, and the professional mask slides back on. I have a photograph of me as a child, arms crossed with a defiant look on my face. I don't recall why, but I remember it floated into my consciousness at the time, making me smile, dissipating some of the irritation.

I am reminded of a sentence: 'an experience is not an isolated event; it is always a historical event placed within the unfolding autobiography of the person's life experience' (Johns 2004b: 4). However, I did stop myself moving into child mode to my manager's demand. I pressed the pause button and reframed the moment. The idea of *reframing* is changing the way we think about something – shifting from the back foot to the front foot.[2]

I gather my composure and pursue what I need to do in face of the ceaseless demand and later, when I'm ready, I go to the general ward and assess the lady. She fell at home and broke her hip. The surgical team had agreed with her family that she would be at further risk if she returns home. Now she waits for placement in a residential home. Apparently she was low in mood and confused at times. After my assessment I inform my manager that the woman felt low in mood because she felt that going into a home meant she was going to die there and her life had ended. The only evidence of confusion was that she didn't know what day it was. I rationalise this away, knowing how easy it is to lose track of time in hospital. Therefore, in my opinion she does not have a mental health issue that warrants admission. The silence at the other end of the phone says more than words. You know that feeling when you say something to someone and it isn't what they want to hear?

A couple of hours later I am informed that the lady in question is being admitted to us. Expletives of exasperation litter my journal.

Showdown. I confront my manager. I argue that the lady would now have the stigma of a psychiatric label. Mental health problems in the older person are both negative and prevalent in society (Stokes 1992). She silences me, telling me that the 'powers that be' had put pressure on her to admit the lady. I try to assert the ethical perspective but my voice has no power. I am reminded of knowing my place.

The agenda is about 'bed blocking and waiting lists' not the plight of a single woman. The stark truth is that the transactional organisation is first and foremost concerned with its own smooth running (Freidson 1970). Silencing myself is also a reflection of smooth running – to silence my voice of dissent in case I scratch the smooth surface. In an effort to transcend the brewing conflict, I focus on how we can care for the lady. We do have beds available, and for all I knew that bed was needed for someone in dire need. It didn't entirely remove my concern for the person ending up on a psychiatric ward when there is no need. That is reinforced when my manager says, 'It's down to system failure and if that had not occurred she wouldn't have come to us.' Systems failure is the scourge of the transactional organisation.

Systems, as Senge (1990) points out, can only be understood by contemplating the whole and not just an individual part. I appreciate that the system clogs up, beds need to be found for those in more need and I do want to collaborate with my general nursing colleagues, but what angers me is the way in which it's done. My vision differs from *theirs* (*them and us* language that is hardly collaborative).

How could I have responded more effectively as a leader? Could I be more assertive? Perhaps the assertiveness action ladder would guide me. (Table 4.1). Okay, let's climb it.

I stumble on the fourth rung – 'being able to make a good argument'. And yet my argument seemed reasonable. I took the moral ground but was rebuffed. I trip on the ninth rung – 'keeping self and other in "adult" mode'. My manager was transmitting the hierarchical anxiety down to me. I tried not to revert to child mode yet withered as her demand (anxiety) grew in response to my defiance. However, I was mindful of this dynamic.

The tenth rung – *yielding* is not failure. Yielding is retreating with my integrity intact knowing I have done my best. Service is about letting go of ego. Servant leaders are warriors prepared to enter the political arena and facilitate the organisation to move towards a more equitable system, capturing the broader issues of social justice and improve patients' lives and health. If I had stuck to my guns could it have been different?

10	Being able to tread the 'fine line' of pushing an issue and yielding	(the controlled self)
9	Keeping self and other in 'adult' mode	(the managed self)
8	Being adept at counter-coercive tactics against more powerful others	(the empowered self)
7	Being adept at interaction skills	(the skill to assert self)
6	'Taking the plunge'	(the resolve to assert self)
5	Creating the optimum conditions to maximise effectiveness	(the scheming self)
4	Being able to make a good argument	(the knowledge to assert self)
3	Understanding the boundaries of autonomy and authority in role	(the right to assert self)
2	Having a focused vision for practice	(the ethic to assert self)
1	Having the felt need to assert self	(the motivational self)

Table 4.1 The assertive action ladder

Source: Johns 2009

Positioning myself within the Thomas-Kilmann conflict mode instrument (see Figure 4.1), I had endeavoured to be collaborative and yet felt pushed into a competitive mode. Competition is where two people struggle to 'win' the situation, often driven by personal agendas. It can become a power game with winners and losers. I didn't want to lose but yielded to accommodate my manger's insistent demand, at least for this moment. Before, I might well have been tearful, an emotional mess – the beaten child, angry, resentful and hurt. My ethical stance was not heard, my professional opinion discounted. Do I imagine that I really had a say in the decision-making over this woman's transfer? I may have gained an understanding but still it makes me feel like a very small cog in a huge machine. Resisting my manager was not easy because of the authoritative nature of transactional power with its underlying threat of sanction. This is such an insight because I realise I do this with my own staff. This form of power is thrown from above but I rarely see who's throwing it. Perhaps this is the problem! The most significant lesson is to remember my feelings of being disempowered and devalued. If I cannot make a chink in the organisational armour above, I can ensure I am more mindful of the way in which I treat others. That requires broad shoulders and I need the support of my staff to shoulder it. Then 'we' can shoulder it.

The Thomas and Kilmann conflict mode instrument (1974) offers me, as a leader, a pragmatic tool in which to position my conflict management mode

Assertive

Competition		Collaboration
	Compromise	
Avoidance		Accommodation

Non-cooperative

Cooperative

Non-assertive

Figure 4.1 Conflict mode instrument

Source: Thomas and Kilmann 1974

> The instrument enables the leader to position her conflict response style within the grid to view the tension between her desired response (collaboration is always the intended mode of leadership) and actual response. It enables the leader to reflect on the nature of this tension and what she needs to do to move towards collaboration.

within the particular situation. I have used the tool many times, given the number of conflict situations I face on a daily basis. It helps me be mindful of my conflict mode position and my intention to be in collaborative mode in tune with my leadership values. However, this requires the ability to transcend personal agendas and stay in adult mode. However, it takes two to tango, and thus being collaborative is difficult when others, notably those in senior management, do not want to play this game. However I am mindful enough to see that my effort to be collaborative is viewed as threats to their authority and makes them feel uneasy.

Thomas and Kilmann note the value of different modes under diverse circumstances. However, I consider that adopting other modes besides collaboration must be deliberative for good reason rather than a subconscious reaction to emotional tension. I resonate with Cavanagh's (1991) observation that my predominant learnt styles of managing conflict had been avoidance and accommodation. However, I can be a feisty, tough competitor if my cage is really rattled but then, no doubt, I would be labelled as emotional. Compromise is never a satisfactory position because it rarely leads to the best decision because one person's agenda or power is always the greater.

Reflection exposes my linear thinking, the way I seem to take everything on face value with no questioning my practice or that of others. Wheatley (1999) suggests that we need to see the world anew and abandon our Newtonian image of the mechanical world. Easier said than done. I am no spring chicken; social and cultural practices are deeply engrained in my practice, some of which I am not even aware of! Reflection allows these insights to emerge, however painful (Johns 2013). Becoming aware brings further disharmony as I unearth the contradictions between my practice and the reality I find myself in. The power struggle within this experience fuelled my resentment. Maybe now, I can let go of this resentment through seeing the bigger picture.

Like a fairy tale, the story ended happily for the woman – the pawn in the political game. The community nursing team and social services felt they could support this woman in her own home. A package of care was put in place and she was discharged, much to her delight. Perhaps that was only possible because she was housed with us. Most of all I remember the kindness of the person who brought me tea and my genuine appreciation. That thought lifts me.

Beatrice

Some months later. Beatrice has been on the ward for a few months. She is a D-grade staff nurse. She works in a calm manner, quietly competent; nothing seems to faze her. Tom, a senior staff nurse, is assigned to support her development. He informs me that Beatrice wants promotion to an E grade, which would normally be expected, and he is helping her to achieve this. However, I have heard some worrying concerns through the *shadow system*. When asked if she would do something, she replied, 'I am not doing that. It is not my job. The senior staff should do it. I've been here long enough, I should get the E grade.'

Other staff are unhappy with her attitude and have confronted her. However, she is resolute in not changing her attitude. It's hard to believe that someone who wants promotion would say these things. I assume that if you want promotion then surely you would show that you are capable. As a consequence my impression of Beatrice shifts dramatically. Now I see her as lazy and difficult – not good labels to apply.

I challenge myself: 'How should I tackle this?' Do I come down with all my authoritative guns blazing and confront her or do I avoid the conflict and hope it goes away? The old ways are tugging at me but the curious child within keeps turning the pebble over. I reject both ways.

Being mindful, I suspend my assumption of her being lazy to explore her perspective. I decide to offer Beatrice clinical supervision as a forum to explore this issue. Clinical supervision is an established system on the ward to enable staff development. Paramount to effective supervision is for the supervisor to be non-judgemental (Johns 2013). Beatrice agrees and we arrange an appointment. My mind is set on fostering an adult–adult relationship, but perhaps I am not so un-judgemental as she responds defensively, resulting in a temper tantrum. Instinctively I recognise she views what I regard as an opportunity as an attack on her integrity. How do I turn this around? I know I mustn't react like a parent trying to quell her temper.

I invite her to share her feelings and thoughts. It helps. She wipes away her tears as I listen. She shares her world view, which centres around her culture. She is from an African background and holds deeply ingrained hierarchical views. Her nursing socialisation process was that each nursing grade had a rigid boundary that one did not cross. She did not have a counterpart of the same grade on the ward to compare herself with, so she was relying upon her personal map. Perhaps she feels oppressed, which, as Roberts (2000) suggests, manifests itself as passive aggression. Cope (2001) discusses the concept of mental maps, which are unique and assist in making sense of the world. Sharing my map helps Beatrice reveal her own. We identify a shared map to enable us to move forward.

We examine the job descriptions of the D and E grades. There is only one difference: that D grades do not work nights. Beatrice felt she's capable but hadn't been given the opportunity to do this. So we plan the off-duty for her to achieve this, working with another staff nurse to guide her. She also identifies an area of interest that she would like to lead on – being the ward's contact for the Black Minority Ethnic Group. My negative attitude dissipates. I feel positive towards her. I recognise how judgemental I had been without appreciating her position. Now I open a space where we can dwell together in common endeavour. My concern is for her growth, not for my control, and yet, paradoxically, I am now more in control through letting it go. My ego is still pushing at me yet I can contain it.

A deeper insight emerged as I tried to understand my internal unease of being a manager and leader. I recognised that moving from nurse to manager is a difficult transition. In a way it's a sense of loss, no longer being part of the 'club', set apart, my clinical-caring self put on a shelf, as I was given a new set of powers – the root of my distrust; I had lost or forgotten the connection to others. In its place, I found I was fulfilling the organisational expectation to perpetuate the paternalistic management role. I clearly saw I was not prepared, and probably never had been, for leadership.

However, I have found that two children examining the pebbles on the shore are better than one. The reconnection process confirms that my lost sense of caring has been in part due to the loss of connection. Now I can recover caring, sublimating clinical caring into leadership caring. I feel a sense of liberation, as if I have burst free from shackles or emerged from Plato's cave to see a whole new world beyond the harping parental flames that licked my skin and caused me anguish.

Moving on

We are eighteen months into the leadership programme. I say 'we' because of my connection to the other leaders within this leadership community. I feel a security in being part of a greater whole. I have been introduced to a variety of philosophies, models of change management, the concept of resistance and strategies in managing conflict. I have grown more aware of the power discourses within the organisation as the rebellion within me grew. And yet I am now more frustrated and disillusioned with my professional life than I was at the beginning of the course. I fully align with Roberts (2000) who postulated that nurses who return to graduate study often feel unsettled in their jobs. She points out that although fellow classmates offer support and together acknowledge the conflict, returning to the work environment only serves to highlight the contradiction. I sit in the group thinking servant leadership is a wonderful ideology but very difficult to put into practice.

More conflict

A critical point came just after writing an assignment on chaos theory.[3] This had enabled me to explore the relationship between leadership and chaos theory. Chaos theory recognises the inherent order that patterns around meaning within the apparent chaotic nature of everyday practice. It is about seeing the whole picture and the way things relate within the whole. I could see by holding to my leadership values I could be more in control than with my previous reactive responses. Indeed, I can recognise that the more I had previously grasped at control, the more things slipped away from me, demanding even greater control. With leadership, I slacken the reins rather than hold them tighter.

We have appointed Ivy as a new clinical team leader. In-house conflict had historically been encountered, but the magnitude of conflict and chaos that the team leader brought was something extraordinary. In response, I guided her to adopt a similar leadership perspective. It seemed to work.

Inside a few weeks we had overcome many conflicts and things seemed to have settled down. I felt secure in the knowledge that the ward was in safe hands whilst I went on holiday.

Nearly three weeks later, with a wonderful tan, relaxed and energised, I came back to face a holocaust. My learning had not prepared me for this chaos. I doubted whether any of the espoused, advocated literature and teachings were of any worth. I doubted my leadership and questioned where I had gone wrong. I asked myself, 'Is this struggle worth it?' The worst thing was my self-blame. I struggle with guilt at the best of times. It is a parental trait. I trusted my children to be responsible when I was on holiday and they failed me. Now I feel anxious and resort to berating them as before.

So what happened?

The storm I returned to was verging on a tempest, the staff at the point of throwing themselves overboard in the raging seas rather than stay afloat with the 'she devil' who had assumed the role of captain in my absence. The staff had likened her to a 'little Hitler' with her parades, uniforms, order and complete power. I had staff threatening to leave. I had staff not speaking to her. I had staff believing I had betrayed them.

Ivy said, 'I'm glad you're back.'

I wasn't! She believed it was all the staff's fault that they had been obstructive and had sabotaged her efforts and deliberately thwarted her instructions. As this was affecting three-quarters of the team, I felt that, despite my new learning, I had to resort to command and control tactics to reassert order. I listened to the staff's woes culminating in a report that I sent to my manager. The system then took over, much to my relief. Ivy was removed from clinical practice. I had let my parents take charge. The huge weight around me lifted. But I am left with a nagging doubt. The flames in the cave mock my leadership aspirations. Yet the crisis was urgent.

To be a servant leader is to respond in terms of what is best for the whole, even if one person is sacrificed. I had tried to prepare Ivy for leading the team but it had not worked. The staff saw me as a heroine in slaying the 'she devil'. My managers see me as decisive. I win both ways. So why do I beat myself up about this? Because I let my anxiety get the better of me. I judge myself harshly.

I could have given up the course. Why didn't I? My father always said I was 'stubborn'. I agree with that, and that stubbornness helps me persevere.

Another insight emerged that what may seem negative can also be positive. Were my and Ivy's leadership styles poles apart? Possibly by letting go of the reins I went too far. Maybe I became 'laissez-faire' in my leadership?

Perhaps I hadn't explained my new vision of leadership to my colleagues. Mental maps adrift, disconnection again. I let chaos into my life, yet paradoxically through the chaos creativity emerged. Had the staff, over the month without recognising it, sucked up some of the new leadership qualities I was trying to implement? Was this why there was such a stark contrast in my and Ivy's leadership? If this assumption is correct, then it would suggest that the team had been feeling empowered and resented it being taken away.

In the community of inquiry, it is suggested that when we let go of the reins, staff can run around like children and view it as a lack of leadership. With hindsight, if I had shared my servant leadership vision more explicitly and involved staff in this vision, then perhaps there would have been less misunderstanding. I had seen leadership as *my* journey, not a *collective* staff journey. My colleagues confirmed my assumption. They appreciated my new leadership and resented Ivy's undermining authoritarian approach. They had not realised this shift in my leadership until the power struggle and conflict emerged. Just a few pebbles now left in my pocket.

Beyond games and giggles

Mark and I are having a giggle. He's recounting a story that happened yesterday. He answered the phone in the staff office and found himself having a bizarre conversation with someone who wanted the police. It was several minutes into the conversation before he realised that a patient had picked up the phone in the reception and dialled the staff office extension. We were enjoying the humour of it when Rose, a staff nurse, interrupted and broke the bubble. Rose is not a nurse whom I would call lighthearted. She is a rather serious person who rarely sees humour in a situation. She evokes in me a feeling of being caught out. The same feeling I got at school when the teacher admonished us for giggling in class. I am feeling guilty again for laughing in the serious world of nursing. She rants about the consultant and community staff. The consultant had decided to discharge a patient, and although a package of care had been set up, Rose was anxious that the patient won't be able to cope. She feels that due to his mobility problems he may fall. She also feels that no one is listening to her. The consultant follows her in and joins the heated debate by accusing Rose of undermining her authority and decision. The phone rings. It is the community nurse asking what's going on. He's been told different stories by both concerned and now doesn't know whether to continue the arrangements or not. Mark rolls his eyes upwards, indicating his exasperation at the whole scenario. Conflict of values, perception and authority mixed into a thick soup boiling over, making a mess.

I am in the middle, saying nothing. I feel distinctly detached as if watching the drama from above but knowing that I'm expected to resolve the situation. Be mindful, is the message that floats out of the ether. I suddenly feel very calm, as if I have transcended the conflict. Chaos has a way of self-organising.

The others must have noticed, for it had a calming effect on them. I sense that one's calmness can radiate to others; pure chaos theory, whereby one's small actions, like smiling instead of frowning can have a profound effect upon others. It is hard to hold anger when smiling. I read that somewhere but cannot put my finger on it. And yet I *was* irritated by their behaviour. It rippled through me like a wave gathering momentum. I recognised my risk of shifting into my 'critical parent' state often triggered when I need to ensure the unit runs smoothly. It is an anxiety transmitted through the hierarchical system that continues to infect me when under severe strain. Where does my 'critical parent' come from? Is it just my socialisation shaped by organisational patterns or does it go even deeper in my childhood roots? I view my childhood as being relatively free from parental rule. I was a very independent child, my parents allowing a liberal freedom. Berne (1964) postulates that people make decisions in childhood that shape the rest of their lives. This was not a gradual realisation but one that just hit me (eureka) when I was in the bath. I was a shared child between my parents and grandparents, spending as much time with both. I had a double dosing of parental guidance! I preferred being in the company of adults. When adults act as children it annoys me, bringing out my critical parent. I apologise for sidetracking, but this has been an utter revelation that helps me understand where I have come from. I can see myself reflexively (Johns 2013) which liberates me to move forward.

I resist the demand of my critical parent and open a space for dialogue, listening and appreciating their respective positions in terms of the patient's best interests. Empathic listening reveals the mind maps of others in order to see the world as they view it (Cope 2001). Perhaps then these competitive practitioners can set aside their own interests so the conflict can best be resolved.

The consultant always takes the high ground so Rose's resistance or competitive style with the consultant is helpful because it exposes real tensions of authority within the multidisciplinary team. Rose's refusal to lie down and be submissive to medical authority is a mark of her integrity when she feels the patient's best interests are in jeopardy. She refuses to play the submissive role. Indeed, Rose can be difficult to manage from my old transactional perspective because she is not submissive and conforming. Rose tends to use the argument that she is acting in the patient's best interests.

I do sometimes worry, however, that this is not always the case. In this instance, the patient was very clear that he wanted to go home and felt that Rose was preventing this.

Whilst acknowledging Rose's voice and concerns, I draw her attention to the wishes of the patient. I also wondered why Rose was so animated about this particular situation. Was I missing something, something deeper than appeared on the surface? I wondered if Rose had become over involved. She did appear territorial in providing this patient's care. I asked her to justify her position. She admitted she felt protective towards this vulnerable patient but agreed that she had lost sight of the bigger picture. We discussed that, ethically, it would not be the best decision to delay the discharge based upon anxieties that the patient did not share. Rose acknowledged that the patient's demand for autonomy was more significant than the risk he might fall.

Through dialogue we cut a path through the power and ethical discourses to reach a consensus. Dialogue *is* the discipline of team learning. The consultant appreciated Rose's concern for the patient. Winners all around, no shame, no blame. It is possible to create better worlds through servant leadership. The conflict abated, we were able to discharge the patient. We all grow as a consequence.

My leadership felt natural. I genuinely felt I was of service to help these two people resolve their conflict. Listening is opening perspectives, noting unhelpful attitudes, clarifying thinking, reinforcing shared values.

Afterwards, Mark said, 'I liked the way you reinforced the vision.'

I wasn't aware that I had. Another revelation. Leadership has become a part of me without my recognition and, as such, I was transferring it, unconsciously, to my staff. I recognise the brittleness of transactional leadership and the strength of servant leadership.

Shifting the blame culture

I am sitting quietly in my office sorting through mail and paperwork. In the background, there is the noise of the familiar comings and goings of the ward. Amy, a staff nurse, comes in, sits down on a chair and says, 'I've made a drug error.' I turn to face her. I see the fear in her eyes. I instinctively reach towards her to support her. 'When you feel ready tell me about it.'

The error is a serious one. Knowing that Amy is normally meticulous in her administration of medication, I find it hard to believe. She is usually competent, enthusiastic, reliable and solid. Now she sits before me, pale, distressed and shaking. I feel sick and ask her how she is feeling. She also feels sick.

My nurturing parent instinctively arises in me. A mother may be seen to offer protection, security and care. A mother will always protect her young. It is the human response. Now, Amy needs my compassion, not an analytical deconstruction of the event. That will come later. Amy needs me to be as open as she has been with me. Although Amy is an adult, in her panic, she sat there at a loss as to what she should do. Panic narrows one's field of focus. I instruct Amy what she needs to do. Holyoake (2000) suggests that a *hurt* child needs direction and instruction in order to feel safe. I am cognisant of the drug error procedure even though I do not have past experiences of managing drug errors. Amy fearfully asks, 'What will happen to me?'

Her words say so much about the organisation in which we work. Where does this fear of punishment come from? I sense the power of sanction (French and Raven 1968) and how management of the population is achieved through subtle and pervasive operation of power associated with disciplinary processes. Coercive or sanction power is endemic within the transactional culture. It reminds people to know their place. I strongly sense an institutional pressure to reprimand Amy. Blame and shame culture rears its head. It is seemingly in my blood like a toxin as if I am plugged into a common artery. But I don't reprimand her. She does this well enough to herself. Beating people up is not servant leadership. The posture – how can I help Amy best deal with this situation? The servant leader enables people to take responsibility to learn from errors.

The mantra 'Tough on the issues, soft on the person' appeals to my sense of caring, as a nurse, as a mother and parent, but more importantly as a woman. I agree with Wilber (2001) that women tend to stress embodied personal relationships. My connection with Amy matters. Connection makes everything possible. It is a new common artery forming, replacing the toxin-filled one. I can put a valve on the toxic artery to keep it from poisoning me. Connection is the core of servant leadership in that Amy *knows* I am available to hold her in her despair yet without clouding the issues.

Looking back, I realise that I had not valued genuine connection at the beginning of my journey. My connections had all been transactional and muddied with emotion. Amy contacted all the relevant professionals, family and agencies involved and acted on their advice. I supported her throughout, finishing the medication round and being with her in person. With all this completed, she sat in the staff office looking forlorn. Doubt crept in again. Was there anything I had learnt about leadership and the philosophies that would help Amy in her despair? What words will help ease her discomfort? I turned to what I instinctively felt – sympathy, but not in words. I put my arm around her and she in turn did the same.

Connection resonates with the idea of a spiritual leadership as set out by Bolman and Deal (1995) in their book *Leading with Soul*. I am not a religious person, but the book has helped me to see something more mystical about life. The challenge is to discover the gifts we already have. I choose now to follow this spiritual leadership path. I have touched something deeper within me in the quiet afternoon with Amy. My leadership moves to another level, more passionate yet paradoxically less entangled in emotional tension. It is a liberating sense.

Amy chose to share her 'mistake' with all members of the team. Humility, nor being afraid of others seeing us for who we truly are (Mayeroff 1971), are two such leadership qualities. Now Amy becomes a leader. Only when we can accept our real selves can we be present to lead. She also contacted our lead in pharmacy to provide further education for herself and the team. Senge (1990) believes that learning as a team is vital in a learning organisation. I am surprised and pleased that Amy viewed her experience not as an isolated event but one in which others could learn. The team's response is compassionate. I watch them acting in just the way I had. Perhaps we are all adults, but the parent in us is not so far away when rubbed with anxiety.

I see clearly how my past parental behaviour has been imitated by others. Whether that be good or bad I do not know, but if given the situation again I would respond in a similar way. Bolman and Deal (1995) say perhaps it is better to be a great person than a great leader. Greenleaf would say a great person *is* a great leader.

The patient showed no signs or suffered no ill effect from the miscalculation of medication. She was more concerned that she had become the focus of nursing attention, which she did not like, and told us so in no uncertain terms. I am not even going to contemplate what would have happened if she had become ill. That's a whole different ball game!

Turning IT around

The final turn of my journey. I am now acting modern matron whilst our existing matron is seconded. I still manage the ward with the new responsibilities yet without a new team leader to assist me. I feel exhausted and frazzled. In the role of modern matron I am expected to ensure the cleanliness of the environment. The launch of the Matron's Charter (Department of Health 2004a) sets out criteria for delivering cleaner hospitals, including all staff receiving education in infection control.

I journal:

> **It** lands on my desk. I view it as just another piece of work, that I heap upon my ever-increasing workload of things to do. **It** concerns the training of all staff in infection control and, in particular, the control and prevention of MRSA.

The Department of Health (2002b) recognises the serious national and global problem of MRSA. This training is a computer programme that can be accessed in the work environment. Pratt et al. (1999) argue that implementation programmes are more likely to succeed if located within the structure of the organisation. From a management point of view this is easier than rostering all staff to attend a study day. The initiative not only included nursing personnel but housekeepers and administration staff. I view it as another paper exercise taking up time in an already busy world. Half-heartedly, I completed the online training, printed off the booklet, gave it to all staff to complete in their own time and forgot about it.

Now you would think that after all I have learnt about change management, sharing the vision, team working and evincing a concern for the whole (Schuster 1994); I would have known better. It is no surprise then that apart from a couple of staff no one else completed it.

> Was I committed? No.
> Did I get a kick up the backside? Yes. The toxin artery pumping its venom.
> Did I feel guilty, which manifested itself as resentment? Yes.
> Did I have a childish temper tantrum, consisting of moans like 'They don't understand the workload we have'? Yes.
> Did I do a turnaround and become the servant leader I wish to be? Yes, of course I did.

I felt a sense of injustice. As Paley (2002) argues, when the transactional voice says 'get it done and get it done within a week', it promotes a sense of injustice and childish rebellion inducing the critical parent response with threat of punishment.

As I roll over the pebbles I draw upon the creative child within. How do I move beyond injustice to view this as a positive challenge? Cunningham and Kitson (2000) suggest that challenges require imaginative and committed leadership. So I used my imagination and contacted the lead person, Sarah, in infection control. Sarah informed me that as no team in the trust had completed the course, there was a competition running. Good old-fashioned reward power. Its blatancy made me smile. As I have noted earlier, my transformational inclination has been to move away from authoritative sources of power, namely positional, reward and coercion, to embrace more facilitative sources of power: referent and expert power (French and Raven1968). Sarah's enthusiasm and personality balanced reward power with referent and expert power. Her enthusiasm was infectious, spreading through myself and the team. The implicit transactional threat of coercion or sanction evaporated.

I journal:

> I rise to the challenge. Yet how am I going to achieve this? How am I expected to get twenty plus staff through this course in a week? Stuff the time limit! We'll do it when we can. I'll hold staff meetings to explain what we are being asked to do, keeping my resentment mindfully in check. I feel my resistant child still bubbling under the surface.

My mind turned to change management and change management models. I was attracted to Burnes' (1990) model of nine elements to manage change (see Figure 5.9). The elements of raising awareness, creating a vision and understanding fears were crucial. This brought up the issue of trust again. I had to trust the staff to help me with the task. It had to become *our* task, not just mine. A community task. However, whilst recognising the usefulness of this model in the long term, the pressure from above did not afford the luxury of time.

Trust

A recurring theme through this journey is my difficulty with trusting staff. Rationally, I know leadership is based on thick trust (Cope 2001), so where does my resistance to trust come from? It is no longer good enough to say this without attempting to find the reason. I believe it may be a gender difference. I work back through my life until I'm finally back to my childhood again. At the age of five my parents presented me with twin sisters. My life changed. They reported me to my parents for any misdemeanour and blamed me for acts they did, and thus I learnt not to trust women. Berne (1961) notes how childhood experiences transfer through to adulthood. These feelings are still with me to the present day. To trust the team I have to let go of my childhood angst. The power of reflection to unearth such patterns feels awesome.

I asked the team what resistance they felt towards the training. I did this to surface, understand and confront resistance, to welcome resistance as indicative of collaboration towards shared success. I know that resistance occurs because change is perceived as threatening (Copnell 1997). Some of the team revealed they are not computer literate. In fact our 73-year-old housekeeper has never been near a computer. Yet she responds positively because she felt listened to and valued.

The team heard my cry, 'Come on, guys, cut me some slack. Let's get this done and get them upstairs off our back.' The team responded with vigour and with no resistance. Two weeks later the training was completed. They exceeded my expectations. Result: second in the whole trust. We celebrated our success. We could play and win the transactional game with a smile rather than a frown. Sarah taught me well. I might have said *the proud parent retires with a well-deserved cup of tea*. Now I can say *the servant leader served the tea well*.

Being in the present, every moment is *naturally* a learning opportunity. It is simply the way it is, the nature of servant leadership to serve in the best way with vision, wisdom and compassion, to enable others to grow and become who they need to become. I cannot promise not to dip into my old bag of behaviour or step back into the world from where I came. However I do feel that servant leadership *is* my way of being. I have entered the stream and go with the flow. I have worked towards this and I do not intend to give up the challenge but acknowledge the challenge it remains. But for the moment I have reached saturation point. I need a rest. So I immerse myself in the garden for recuperation. Servant leaders withdraw to keep in good shape to serve well. So many lessons learnt. No more leadership books to read for fear of clogging up the new arteries of leadership. At some point in the future the urge to pick up a pen and resume studying will become a thirst I cannot ignore. My own growth is now in my blood.

The construction of my narrative has taken many twists and turns, demonstrating the complex and changing nature of my daily practice. The penetrative process of unravelling my own thinking and committing reflections to paper has in itself altered my perceptions and created change. I have discovered that challenge is not to be feared, life need not be static and mountains can occasionally move. I invite my readers to ride in tandem with me viewing the moving scenery through the filter of their own experience and applying it to their own lives. I depend on you, the reader, to move the narrative beyond an articulation of personal experience into the realm of wider interpretation and social relevance (Pinar 1981). It is from you that the text gains its validity and movement. Stories can infect perceptions, invade complacency, amplify conscience and change lives.

Conclusion

There is much passion in Alison's narrative. It is as if she has been bitten with the bug of leadership and it has infected her. She recognises the journey is tiring, reflecting on the need for perseverance and support notably from within her own team to complement the support within the community of inquiry. The leader is able to do this through the creation of community. In doing so, her leadership is inculcated through her team.

Reflection

- To what extent do you feel you belong to a community in your practice?
- How might community be developed?
- To what extent do you feel 'of service' to your colleagues and patients?

Notes

1. Referential power – Alison refers to French and Raven's typology of power – see page 102.
2. Shifting from front to back foot – Alison refers to front foot thinking – see Figure 1.6.
3. See Appendix 1 for programme design.

5 Leading Change, Easing Conflict, Quality is the Leader's Business

Alison and Martha's narratives reveal how journeys of becoming a leader are journeys of change from both a personal and organisational perspective. As they explore their new leadership they move into dialogue with others to negotiate and secure their leadership and its inevitable impact on clinical practice and systems that support practice. Put another way, they become change agents. A change agent is someone who is curious, committed and intelligent about practice and ways it can be developed to ensure the most effective care. By curious I mean nothing is taken for granted. By committed I mean my practice really matters to me. By intelligent I mean I am able to see things for what they really are and weigh up the consequences of implementing change. What, on the surface looks a good idea, for example clinical supervision, becomes distorted as it is accommodated within the culture of everyday practice with the consequence that what seemed a good idea has only a limited impact on practice.

The skill of being a successful change agent cannot be assumed, and yet most people approach change without knowledge of change management. Maybe on the surface, change does seem unproblematic but such naivety is a minefield.

Change is a dynamic life force. Without change, things become stagnant, complacent and deteriorate.

Nothing is ever static. Things are always changing. Planned change should always be purposeful to improve quality, and quality is everybody's business.

Leaders continuously evaluate practice:

• Does current practice lead to best care and outcomes for patients, families and staff?

- Are the systems in place to most effectively support the delivery of practice?
- What support and development do staff require?
- Do we utilise our budget most effectively?

As a leader I view change as something positive despite the anxiety and conflict it seems to generate because people do not seem to like change and are naturally motivated to resist it despite any rational appeal. Change is emotional. It always evokes resistance because it always disturbs the status quo. In everyday practice people are motivated to maintain the status quo, a relative state of equilibrium that, if disturbed, creates social unrest because people's interests are threatened, particularly within trans-actional organisations where self-interest and self-preservation may be more important than patient care. People are comfortable with the status quo and hence naturally resist any shift that disrupts their comfort even though the change may rationally lead to an improved quality of patient care. Lewin's (1951) force field analysis offers the change agent a useful approach to plot and view the driving and resisting forces to any change (Figure 5.1).

Klein (1976) sets out a number of considerations regarding managing the status quo (Figure 5.2). As a general rule, the focus for managing change is to reduce the resisting forces on the premise that reinforcing the driving forces will only strengthen the resistance. To limit resistance, two considerations are vital. First, change must be meaningful for those affected by the change. This may prove difficult for people when change is instigated at a senior management level. I imagine the recoil 'What do they know about it?' Indeed, but change that affects systems or the way the organisation is run often happens that way. Systems provide the background for service delivery and are difficult to change at a unit level. In a world flooded with change ideas, it is easy to appreciate why practitioners might become cynical and resist change, especially change imposed on them. Second, those affected by change must be genuinely involved in the change process. Their voices must be heard and respected.

From a positive perspective, resistance to change is useful to the leader because it prompts her to reconsider issues that may not have necessarily

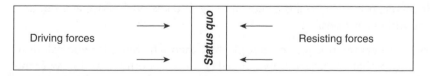

Figure 5.1 Lewin's force field analysis

1.	There is almost a universal tendency to seek to maintain the status quo on the part of those whose needs are being met by it.
2.	Resistance to change increases in proportion to which it is perceived as a threat.
3.	Resistance to change increases in direct response to the pressure of change.
4.	Resistance to change based on fear of the new circumstances is decreased when those involved have the opportunity to experience the new under the conditions of minimal threat.
5.	Temporary alterations in most situations can be brought about by use of direct pressure, but these changes are accompanied by heightened tension and will yield a highly unstable situation.
6.	Commitment to change increases when those involved have the opportunity to participate in the decision to make and implement the change.

Figure 5.2 A number of key factors for the leader to consider in managing resistance (Klein 1976)

been clearly thought through or communicated well enough including her own contribution to resistance. Through dialogue, resistance is mediated. In other words, resistance can be a positive rather than a negative force for the leader (Ford et al. 2008).

Balancing power

Before continuing it is significant to consider power. Martin Luther King Jr's words of wisdom are a good place to begin – *I am not interested in power for power's sake, but I'm interested in power that is moral, that is right and that is good.*[1]

A mantra for the leader! Power is an energy that patterns the environmental field. Power influences behaviour and relationships between people. Aspiring leaders tend to view 'power' as a negative word because they generally perceive power as a controlling force rather than a creative force. However, power in itself is a neutral thing. It takes on positive and negative ions within relationships.

Power operates not just on people but through them. Power relations are those that structure how everyday life will be lived and how forms are produced and reproduced to limit and constrain, as well as contextualise and redefine what one is able to be (Simon and Dippo 1986). In transactional organisations managers twist power to control whereas in transformational organisations leaders use power to stimulate creativity. Control tends to stifle creativity in its demand for conformity, whilst creativity tends to liberate people. The difference is stark and profound. The leadership journey can be seen as the conversion of force to power.

Hawkins (2002: 133) notes, 'The source of power is meaning, the significance of life itself. Force always creates counterforce, its effect is to polarize rather than unify, inevitably leading to win-lose dichotomies with concomitant dependence, creating enemies and is invariably costly.'

The word *force* reflects the negative side of power and a source of oppression (Fay 1987). French and Raven (1968) view leadership power as either authoritative or facilitative (Figure 5.3). Simply put, an emphasis on authoritative power characterises the transactional organisation whereas an emphasis on facilitative power characterises the transformational organisation. Leadership is a strong shift towards an emphasis on facilitative modes of relating whilst diminishing authoritative modes. Living things prefer persuasion to force (Webster 1917). However, positional power is leverage to open a space for the leader to assert his or her influence. Positional power may also be appropriate when people do not take responsibility for their performance, a likely scenario within a transactional culture. Coercive power aligned to positional power creates a toxic environment where people are motivated by fear of sanction. From a transactional perspective, reward is more extrinsic as part of the transactional contract – 'if you do an effective job you will be suitably rewarded.' This type of reward always has a coercive edge to it – 'if you don't do an effective job then I have a stick to beat you with'. Hence reward is conditional.

Authoritative	Facilitative
Positional power: legitimate power given by the person's position within the organisation	Relational power: power of influence that stems from relationships, for example charisma
Coercive power: the power to impose sanction	Expert power: power that stems from knowing
Reward power: extrinsic	Reward power: intrinsic
Transactional	Transformational

Figure 5.3 French and Raven's power modes of relating (1968)

Kelly writes: Humphris (2002) suggests that the command and control style of leadership fails to engage the knowledge and skills of the workforce. For nurses, like myself, who have been in the NHS for many years, this type of 'leadership' has been the norm from our early days as students. Only the brave or foolish broke the rules and dared to question the commands of a more senior nurse even when they thought they could do things better. Wilkinson (1996) suggests that this is common in the health service, as traditionally many health professionals have been groomed to be subservient and take direction from those in higher authority. Humphris (2002) suggests that staff may even feel comfortable with this model of leadership [sic] as they know where the boundaries are and dislike change. It is a parental form of leadership that does not encourage responsibility.

Sanction stunts growth. People become fearful within a blame-and-shame culture. Keep your head down or it will get shot off!

Within a transformational culture reward is primarily intrinsic, for example, the realisation of one's vision or appreciation of good practice. This is not to say extrinsic reward would not be appreciated!

Establishing new power norms takes time, tolerance, patience and investment when power patterns have been embodied and reinforced daily by normal patterns of relating.

Within the transactional organisation, positional power or authority is significant to manage change from a traditional top-down approach whereby those affected by change can easily be excluded or paid minimal lip service with regard to involvement. In contrast, leaders strive to create secure environments for people to enable self-expression without fear of sanction, moving towards a bottom-up inclusive culture.

Fear

The transactional system operates with its fear of sanction. This fear works to keep people in their place. It is endemic, socialised into people through normal patterns of relationship. Through compliance (keeping their head down), people within the transactional culture can opt out and not take responsibility, working at a low level of achievement so long as they do not upset the organisation's smooth running. The hard hand of coercion is counterproductive. The soft hand of the transformational leader is more powerful. As Tzu (1999: 78) says, 'Everyone knows this is true, but few can put it into practice.'

Beck (1997: 61) identifies two types of fear. One kind of fear is ordinary; if physically threatened we react, do something and may run, fight or call the police. But we do something; this is natural, ordinary fear. But most of our anxious life is not based on that but upon false fear. False fear exists because we misuse our mind based on a constant and uneasy evaluation of ourselves and others. This type of fear is a form of ignorance and insecurity, what Schuster (1994) refers to as the dark side of ego where everything gets interpreted in terms of the self rather than for what it really is. Ignorance is not bliss!

> Karen writes: I see how in the past I have traded creativity for compliance; I have had to learn to reposition myself from a reactive to creative standpoint. I know deep down if I am honest with myself about wanting to realise transformational leadership, that this will simply not be possible if I am constantly living in this state of fear.

In praise of authority

Prior to my appointment as senior nurse in two community hospitals I had been a clinical practice facilitator with the remit to develop clinical practice in community hospitals within West Dorset Health Authority. In this role I became increasingly frustrated by my inability to influence the development of clinical practice. Looking back, I can perceive this inability was due to a number of 'resistant' factors (Figure 5.4) that I hadn't appreciated whilst immersed within the situation. Had I been more mindful of myself as a leader, then perhaps I would have appreciated these factors and responded more appropriately. My power of influence was not strong enough within my limited time spans within each individual hospital. As a consequence, I felt that I needed authority for leading practice although, as I was to discover at a later date, even authority may falter against unyielding resistance. My driving forces were limited. Even my enthusiasm may have confronted staff with their own lack of passion, hence people may have felt uncomfortable and, paradoxically, this may have strengthened their resistance. It seems common sense on reflection to appreciate that resistance should be expected where change is likely to affect the comfort and meaning of people's lives. People will find it difficult to focus positively on new ideas and practice if they are concerned with maintaining or regaining some continuity with the past (Marris 1986).

The list of resisting forces is daunting. I can see my own need to accomplish change against those who wished I would go away and leave them in peace. Where there is no culture of change, then change threatens to reveal that existing practice has been somehow unsatisfactory. People respond by

Driving forces for change		Resisting forces for change
• My commitment towards realising holistic practice and development of clinical practice for the benefit of patients and staff. • Pressure on community hospital staff to comply with practice development initiatives (as reflected in my appointment).	Status quo	• My lack of authority as an 'outsider' to the practice teams. • I spoke a different language to clinical staff and had different agendas. • Practitioners' ignorance of 'holistic practice' as both an intellectual and practical idea. • My lack of presence due to limited time available to spend across five hospitals undoubtedly diluted my influence. • Lack of leadership within the clinical areas. • A cultural passivity and apathy of clinical staff towards practice development and change. • My lack of expertise as a change agent. • Lack of active organisational support at both the executive and local hospital level (passive transactional management). • The practice areas' lack of vision of community hospitals' practice (practice was very much task driven rather than value driven). • My emphasis on outcome rather than process (given the limited time available and reliance on local 'leaders' to facilitate the change). • My passion was a turn-off for staff because it confronted them with their apathy. • My expectation of the pace of the change.

Figure 5.4 Driving and resisting forces to change

digging in, manning the trenches against the enemy. Yet they had to play along to some extent because of an unstated fear of managerial sanction if they didn't. A frustrating game was being played until I decided I needed the authority of my own practice to instigate change.

Apathy

Perhaps the most insidious resisting factor to change is the apathy of people with whom the leader needs to collaborate with in the change process. To counter apathy, the leader must stir staff commitment and responsibility and encourage them to realise that practice is important and to engage in change is an aspect of professional practice. Yet it is a headache as to how best to engage such people when apathy is rife. The most obvious driving force is to improve patient care. Few staff can deny the veracity of this motive despite their apathy. Hence the value of exploring meaning and creating vision to help staff reconnect to caring, and infuse commitment. As a leader I am driven by a commitment to patient care. I assume and expect all staff would share this commitment. If not, why are they working in health care? Commitment is the bottom line and yet, for many reasons, people may be tired and burnt out, where their commitment is a tiny spark rather than a roaring furnace. One obvious reason is the transactional organisation's failure to recognise the humanness of caring that results in staff not feeling acknowledged and valued. They have become cogs in the machine. They are whipped by slogans such as 'more for less' in response to financial pressures. As we have seen in the media in places like Mid Staffs such mentality results in outrage at poor care. Failed leadership! The first thing a leader must do is to see and respond to people in their humanness.

Senge (1990) outlines a commitment to apathy scale (Figure 5.5) that is useful for the leader to frame and confront people's attitudes. If staff say, 'Yes, I am committed', then the leader can remind them of this fact as necessary. If they say they are not, then it can be explored. Of course they might say 'yes' but mean 'no'! They might seem enthusiastic to your face and then undermine you behind your back.

Leaving West Dorset I was appointed as senior nurse at Brackley Cottage Hospital. The hospital had undergone significant upheaval with the recent closure of its maternity unit. The previous matron had retired after twenty-five years. Midwifery care was transferred to the district general hospital. Midwives could transfer if they wished. One senior midwife chose to remain behind. With the demise of maternity, the hospital now catered for generally elderly people under the care of local GP practices. Morale was low. The hospital was the fiefdom of the senior partner of the GP practice situated across the road. I can remember his loud voice shouting 'Johns!' as he

Commitment	Wants it. Will make it happen. Creates whatever laws/structures are needed.
Enrolment	Wants it. Will do whatever can be done within the spirit of the 'law'.
Genuine compliance	Sees the benefit. Does everything expected and more. Follows 'letter of the law'. Good soldier.
Formal compliance	On the whole sees the benefit. Does what's expected but no more. 'Pretty good soldier'.
Grudging compliance	Does not see the benefit. But also does not want to incur sanction. Does enough of what's expected because she has to, but also lets it be known that she is not really on board.
Non-compliance	Does not see the benefit and will not do what's expected. 'I won't do it and you can't make me'.
Apathy	Neither for or against. No interest or energy – 'Is it 5 o'clock yet?'

Figure 5.5 Commitment to apathy scale (Senge 1990)

confronted me with yet another complaint regarding the management of his hospital. I know that old ways do not shift easily especially when they are grounded in a tradition of domination and subservience.

Leadership at its core is relational. It works through thick trust. 'Trust is the oil that lubricates relationships' (Cope 2001: 152). My leadership priority was to develop trust with practitioners who naturally viewed me with caution, especially as it must have seemed that I had breezed in on my broom, full of new ideas, knocking down and sweeping out the debris of old systems. My background in community hospitals at least gave me some credibility in the sense staff could not reject me in terms of not understanding the nature and culture of community hospitals. In this respect I had 'expert power' alongside my 'authoritative power' of being the senior nurse. Aware of French and Raven's work, my leadership approach was to use facilitative sources of power built upon my positional power – a delicate balance as I worked hard to keep my frustration at bay.

All change needs to be framed within *meaning*. Meaning is the most powerful 'strange attractor', around which order inherently patterns (Wheatley 1999). In other words it gives purpose and direction to practice when held intentionally. Without the group being genuinely signed up to meaning or vision, change will always struggle to take hold. As such, the first quest was to develop a shared vision of practice grounded in patient care in language they understood and valued. New language around primary nursing could be filtered in. Torbert (1978) describes this as social ju-jitsu – talking to people simultaneously in a language they understand whilst addressing to them in a way that undermines the old understandable language and introduces them to a new, more desirable language.

Perhaps, for the first time, practitioners were asked:

'What is care?'

'What does a community hospital exist to do?'

'What did the local community expect from us?'

Responding to these questions gave practitioners a voice to articulate and explore *meaning* as a team. It gave them ownership and responsibility, breaking the rigid hierarchical grip that had existed before my arrival. In response we developed a shared vision of nursing, tailor made for the community hospital, written in a layman's language and included in the patient's information booklet (Johns 1996).

I knew that I must avoid coercive behaviour because of the messages it would give, as if revealing the true tyrant underneath a facade of collaboration. I was bending the tight, straight lines of the transactional culture that worked as a kind of straightjacket into a transformational learning curve. As a leader I was mindful of leading by example by having a strong clinical presence.

The card up my sleeve so to speak was to introduce primary nursing. This decision was not negotiable although how to implement it effectively became the focus for dialogue and consensus. It was certainly 'in vogue' and viewed as the ultimate professional nursing model evolving from task-focused nursing, individual patient care and team nursing. Primary nursing is based around the idea of 'primary nurses' managing a caseload of patients for which they have 24-hour accountability (Manthey 1980). When not on duty, associate nurses continue care as planned by the primary nurse yet with discretion to amend care as appropriate in response to the patient's changing circumstances. Primary nurses act as associate nurses for their colleagues, enabling a cross fertilisation of practice.

Lessons learnt from West Dorset rang bells. To help frame the change process I utilised Ottaway's framework of change as a social process of moving from one set of norms to a new set of norms (1976) (Figure 5.6). Change always requires attention to social norms that govern everyday practice simply because change inevitably disrupts these and creates resistance. Hence the leader is advised to view change as moving from one set

- Contracting the change with followers, thus actively involving the followers in each stage of the change process. This gives ownership and opens patterns of communication. It demands that practitioners take responsibility for their own and collective practice.

- Generating felt need for the change. This is particularly pertinent in an era when health care is bombarded with change that does little to improve the lives of staff and patients, resulting in skepticism at best and cynicism and passive resistance at worst. Felt need is keeping the vision alive, that the change can be viewed within the broader scope of benefitting patient care.

- 'Tailor making' the change to suit the particular circumstance. In this way the leader and followers pay attention to the social norms that govern everyday practice ensuring that the change is most likely to succeed. It is not simply a question of importing an idea and expecting it to work in the knowledge that ideas become distorted to fit existing norms when accommodated into practice. As such, to make something work, social norms need to be adjusted – for example, leadership.

- Piloting the site – so that people can test the change for its value before implementation on a wide scale. This enables people to more objectively assess the value of the change and identify where systems need to be further developed to robustly support it.

- Evaluating the change, that clearly demonstrating its value for wider dissemination.

Figure 5.6 Ottaway's social process approach

of social norms to another. Ottaway's approach to change is congruent with the values of leadership with its emphasis on collaboration, purpose and process. From feedback, I learnt the previous senior nurse/matron had been authoritarian – what she said went. Clearly my style was radically different from what people had previously experienced. Put another way – I was culture shock!

Most change I had experienced working within NHS organisations had been top-down: imposed despite consensus exercises that created an illusion of listening to staff – the 'velvet-gloved' democratic process hiding the 'steel fist' of authority. This is the transactional way. Staff had learnt that much organisational change has little impact on patient care. It was as if change was for change's sake. No wonder people are generally cynical and resistant, feeling like pawns in a chess game.

The collaborative approach always intends to involve all staff in the change process – it is after all their practice! Whilst that sounds easy it wasn't.

When people are used to authoritarian modes of management, it is not easy for them to participate. Being invited to participate is one thing. Wanting to and constructively participating is quite another, especially when you have embodied being subordinate.

It follows that I needed to be patient, open and authentic, willing to give away power to the group process. However, this approach to change requires followers also to be authentic and responsible as collaborators.

My invitation was on the table.

To help me 'sell' primary nursing I established a staff development pro-gramme, bringing in experts in primary nursing so the staff could hear it from those who had practised it. Hearing it from another voice besides my own seemed to give the idea more credence because it could no longer be ascribed to me and resisted as just my idea. Such seminars opened a gate for dialogue, reinforcing a pattern of communication vital to support a culture of collaboration.

Appreciating power is a core attribute of leadership. Although words like transactional and transformational were not in my vocabulary at this time, I was feeling the tension between a collaborative approach to leadership within the prevailing bureaucratic culture of management that emphasised command and control. I knew that shared success in implementing primary nursing depended on each person taking responsibility for first their own role performance and second that of the wider clinical team. Being asso-ciate nurses to each other's patients drew the primary nurses and the others into a mutual responsibility to work together towards ensuring best practice.

- I planned the implementation of primary nursing with the three prospec-tive primary nurses. Two of the primary nurses were the existing ward sisters and the third a young enthusiastic staff nurse who had a degree in nutrition. A clear pecking order existed between these three nurses that imposed itself in my absence. At first, I thought this pecking order would hinder change but paradoxically it enabled it. The dominating behaviour of the midwife sister led to strife amongst other staff. She became iso-lated. She clung to her old authority as a way of holding onto the past. She was tyrannical as she projected her anger at the health authority onto me as representative of a new order. Yet her resistance made sense and needed to be drawn out and her past midwifery role honoured. She needed to make good the broken connection between what was happen-ing now and the angst before she could look forward to the future with any sense of commitment and optimism (Marris 1986). I could appreciate her predicament and support her through her loss, gradually nurturing trust and collaboration between us.

We chose to organise primary nursing territorially. This was significant for the ex-midwife sister, so she could continue to care for patients in what previously had been maternity beds. This decision enabled a continuity of her practice, which mitigated her sense of loss. Being a primary nurse also enabled her to retain authority for care management. Change must always be pragmatic rather than ideal based on local circumstance. Similarly, change cannot be rushed or forced otherwise social processes will become distorted. Hawkins and Shohet (1989: 53) dramatically make the point: 'a man once saw a butterfly struggling to emerge from its cocoon, too slowly for his taste, so he began to blow on it gently. The warmth of his breath speeded up the process all right. But what emerged was not a butterfly but a creature with mangled wings.' As commonly quoted, 'patience is a virtue' and yet this can be so difficult in the transactional, reactive world driven by targets and short-term solutions.

My leadership role was not to dictate or prescribe patient care but to support and develop the primary nurses and other staff to fulfil their roles most effectively in tune with the hospital's vision for practice.

As such I worked 40 per cent of my time in an associate nurse role, developing and role modelling being an associate nurse. In this way I constantly surveyed the primary nurses' practice yet was always mindful of being facilitative rather than authoritative in my feedback. I needed to trust the primary nurses yet set up feedback systems whereby best practice might be known and realised, through which all practitioners, whether primary nurses or care assistants, took responsibility for their own and collective practice. In response, I established a *standards of care* project, creating the opportunity to formally facilitate dialogue of working together towards realising desirable and effective clinical practice within the available resources. Standards of care offered a systematic approach to practice development and quality of care that was tailor made for practice and owned by practitioners (Johns 1990a, b). Quality became both an individual and collective enterprise. In this way, change became inculcated into culture as a dynamic force. Like spinning plates it needed to be constantly serviced to maintain momentum, in this case to loosen the stabilising bolts that tied the hospital to its past tradition . At the same time it had to enable people to feel secure. It was finding the balance between driving forces for change and restraining forces to ensure stability. Yet inexorably the balance was shifting towards change. Slowly ideas began to coalesce. However, after just months, I left to become the general manger of Burford Community Hospital.

Burford Hospital

Burford had a tradition of practice development through the pioneering work of the clinical practice unit (Pearson 1983). The unit was famous, an icon for the potential of nursing to realise its therapeutic potential. Primary nursing was well established. At least I had thought so. Pearson had left Burford three years previously. A ward sister was holding the status quo. Yet holding the status quo is a slippery slope towards decay. Instead of a vibrant unit I found a burnt-out shell gasping on the last vestiges of the Pearson legacy, confused between the old and the new norms. Pearson was a visionary, charismatic, yet he left a vacuum behind him. Successful leadership ensures that new norms created through change are sustained. Fragile and vulnerable, the new norms need constant gardening to grow robust. I learnt the backdraft of consumed charismatic leadership. Nursing development had withered on the vine.

My first task was to pick the rotting fruit and clean the vine, and then connect with the lived reality of faded fame. I felt the sense of disillusionment – 'we've been here before'. The cynics sharpened their tongues. Through this process I was supported by a small minority of practitioners dedicated to therapeutic nursing. This support was vital so I did not feel alone. My broom was out, sweeping through the hospital floors, leaving no stone unturned. Staff ached, for they had been through this upheaval once before. If we genuinely believe in realising best practice then change must be unremitting. It becomes bearable when we feel the need for change and feel our voices are heard and respected from cleaner to matron, from cook to doctor. Everyone has a significant role to play within the whole working towards realising our shared vision. Such values are vital to surface and make explicit at a time of continuous tension between understanding the reality of current practice and the norms that underpin it, and striving to establish a new set of norms based on realising our vision as a lived reality.

At the core of this activity was my exploration of leadership, notably my role in ensuring that staff take responsibility for ensuring the quality of their own and the unit's collective practice. However, it was more than that. It was also about investing in staff to bring out their full potential so each could flourish to realise our shared vision as a shared reality. However, it was not plain sailing.

Conflict

Inevitably, change creates resistance and conflict at every level of the organisation. So many cans of worms were opened. As Alison outlined in Chapter 4, the Thomas and Kilmann conflict mode instrument (Figure 4.1) is a useful framework to reflect on the way leaders manage conflict. Whilst the tool offers five modes of conflict management – avoidance, accommodation, compromise, competition and collaboration – within the messy world of everyday clinical practice it is not straightforward to simply apply a specific mode. Shades of each mode are always in play reflecting our personality and socialisation. To reiterate Alison's words, *leaders always intend to be collaborative*. Yet forces are continuously pulling us into more passive and aggressive modes.

The harmonious team

Karen, one of the associate nurses, was criticised by the night associate nurse because she had written in the patient notes the patient's complaint at the way the auxiliary nurse had spoken to him – like an angry parent admonishing his demand for attention. She felt Karen had transgressed the rules of the harmonious team (Johns 1992, 2013) whereby first and foremost staff are loyal to each other rather than to the patient. As a consequence, conflict is swept under the surface. The illusion of harmony at all costs must be maintained even as the worms writhe and seethe beneath the smooth surface. The harmonious team was a virus infecting the team culture with false values. I burst the infected wound, yet Karen says she wouldn't reveal issues again. She had been put in her place and learnt that it is better to sacrifice the patient than risk alienation from the group. I took the auxiliary nurse aside and listened to her story. She admitted she was cross at the patient. The confronted naughty child confesses her guilt but she insisted Karen's actions were not acceptable. I became the critical parent in my efforts to guide her to take responsibility and prevent warfare through diplomacy. Yet it was hard to see Karen suffer when she tries so hard. She was so vulnerable that I wanted to cradle her like a nurturing parent. She must learn to stand her ground and not be buffeted by the harsh condemning tongues of the furtive subculture that sought to revert to old norms. With collaborative intent, we debriefed at a staff meeting, bringing the dirt into the open so we could clean it properly rather than sweep the emotional mess under the carpet where it would have festered. Being a natural conflict avoider, this was my own tough learning curve – to face conflict head on rather than skirt around the edges. Having a strong vision of self as leader gave me confidence and nurtured my courage to act and role model to others that collaboration must prevail. Karen had reported the issue to Roger, the primary nurse. He had avoided it. Ideally he should have dealt with it but like most nurses (Cavanagh 1991) he also was a conflict avoider. He agreed he should have taken action but felt afraid of stirring the hornet's nest. Lessons for us all.

Mike

Mike was one of the local GPs who managed the medical care of patients at the hospital. He wanted to admit from home a woman dying of cancer for terminal care. I informed him that I had no available beds. He responded by saying there was one empty bed. I explained it was for Mr Collins, a booked admission for the next day for respite care. Mrs Collins was going on a much-needed holiday. The bed was one of two dedicated beds set aside for this purpose. Mike appreciated this but insisted his patient's need had greater priority. Mr Collins would have to lose the bed. I refused. He insisted and still I refused. He stormed off and arranged the woman's admission to the local hospice twenty miles away in Oxford.

Most of the staff supported me but a couple of voices were critical. They felt the doctor should take responsibility for the beds. Perhaps I could have avoided conflict by accommodating Mike's 'demand' but in doing so my authority would have been shredded and my responsibility to Mrs Collins broken. I would have felt very guilty despite the dying woman's real need.

Locked in competitive mode, I was caught on the back foot, in a defensive mode that oppressed me. There are winners and losers. It becomes more than the patients. It becomes an issue of authority. I did not like this style. It left a bad taste in the mouth. We needed to collaborate yet I felt forced into competition because of Mike's own competitive and dominant nature.

Prior to this situation, I generally accommodated the GPs demands, conforming to the natural dominance between doctor and nurse, wary of any 'hell to pay' when this natural professional dominance was transgressed (Stein 1967). However, within this situation, driven by a sense of responsibility, I moved first into collaborative mode and, when this failed, into competitive mode. From a leadership perspective, collaboration is always the intended style. This understanding enabled me to reflect on the nature of this tension to consider what I needed to do to move towards collaboration.[2]

Leadership is moral. What would have been the best decision to make? Who had the greater need? Such ethics are complex. These are the messy swampy lowlands of practice where problems have no easy solutions (Schön 1987). There are no prescriptions. Practice is essentially chaotic guided by our values.

Two days later I made an appointment to see Mike. I said we needed to work collaboratively for the benefit of our local community. He said he had been a GP in the town for ten years and was a better judge of the situation than me and that nursing development ideas were ludicrous. I knew he was trying to put me in my place, to reassert the traditional dominance. But I held my ground and said I was sorry he took that attitude. I had gathered my strength and responded in tune with my collaborative values. No one said that becoming a leader was going to be easy. Old demons of professional dominance haunted me, making me doubt myself. I hung on to my self-esteem by the coat tails. But I needed my closest nursing colleagues to support me. I could not do this alone. Leadership is confident with a strong self-esteem. Mine was challenged. Actions have consequences. Mike did not speak to me for nearly a year. Then at Christmas, softened by wine, the storm passed. Leaders must be resilient and able to ride out storms.

Roger's lament

A few weeks later another incident occured to test my leadership. Luke, one of Mike's GP partners, criticised Mr Waterman's discharge. He felt that the hospital had failed to set up adequate support services for Mr Waterman in the community. This came to light when he visited the family at home. He informed me by letter of his concern. The letter was copied to the director of nursing for the community trust. Stella was new on the patch. She had a reputation for being tough and unequivocal on issues. It was said 'You don't mess with her'. The power of labels. I felt her intimidation when I had recently attended a briefing session where she had outlined her vision and plans for developing clinical services in line with efficiency savings. The corporate squeeze. I had wanted to say something about 'our' vision and 'plans' but something caught my tongue. My voice silenced. She had invited comment but something in her manner warned me to be careful, especially in the public arena. Later I felt angry at myself for not voicing my concern at her proposals. I wonder why we were all so quiet? Do we exhibit oppressed group behaviour? Roberts (1983, 2000) argues that to be empowered and free from oppression one has to become more esteemed in oneself and within a group. This means looking at internalised beliefs about our own inferiority and cycles of self-hatred. Such oppressed groups simply cannot unite to fight against more powerful groups, and hence develop passive–aggressive approaches such as moaning behind the scenes and horizontal violence. I could feel the weight of Stella's positional power and its associated coercive threat steeped in transactional ways of relating. I recognised this point, having shadowed the previous director at trust board meetings, where she was passive in the face of the insistent male chief executive. This pattern of communication is replicated at every level of the transactional hierarchy. Could I break this pattern?

The phone rang. It was Stella's secretary. She wanted to make an appointment for Stella to visit. I sense my fear leak along the edge of my poise. I feel as if I have transgressed and disturbed the smooth running. The insidious nature of coercive power runs deep within my veins. An appointment made for seven days time. No messing about. Stella came on the phone. She wanted me to fax her a report concerning the incident in good time before we met. I immediately want to talk with Leslie, the primary nurse responsible for Mr Watermon's discharge. He was not on duty. I sense the way I transmitted my anxiety down the bureaucratic hierarchy. I wanted to pass it on – pass the buck. Instead I was left with it – institutional angst. Now I could appreciate Nelson Mandela's words: 'It is better to lead from behind and to put others in front, especially when you celebrate victory when nice things occur. You take the front line when there is danger. Then people will appreciate your leadership.'

The next day I cornered Leslie. He was busy with a heavy patient load. He wanted to talk through the situation in his clinical supervision session with me that afternoon. He expressed his frustration. He accepted responsibility for the discharge. He hadn't contacted social services in good time to make continuing care arrangements and forgot to inform the district nurse Mr Waterman was being discharged. He squirmed in his chair. It was not easy for him to accept he had failed. I had no intention of blaming Leslie. I asked what we could learn from this situation and what his response to the GP and family should be. He felt he needed a checklist, and should get the approval of the GP that all was in order prior to discharge. He said he would talk to the GP and write to the family and apologise for the poor discharge.

I responded, 'Okay, Leslie, do it. Draft me a summary of the situation and your intended action.'

Leslie went to see the GP to apologise. Afterwards he said his apology was accepted. It was painful to see Leslie brought to heel, his tail between his legs. He had been put in his place. It was not a place I wanted the primary nurses to be in. I need them to be assertive. I suggested we debrief with the whole team at a later date.

Five days later, I sat with Stella in my small office. I set out the situation and actions taken. Unknown to me she had visited the GP surgery next door to the hospital and spoken with Luke. Luke was satisfied with the actions taken but insisted that care needed to be improved at the hospital. I felt this was a barb thrown at me because of the Mike incident. Hunting in packs. Stella appreciated the nature of primary nursing but insisted that I took a more supervisory role to prevent it from happening again. I felt uncomfortable because I am mindful of a choice – do I meekly accept the censure and agree or do I hold my ground and support our primary nursing values? Clearly our practice needed to be safe and indeed we had no previous complaint. I had every confidence in Leslie's ability. Indeed he was a fine nurse. He had clinical supervision with me and we also met at the standards group to ensure quality. I asserted that the situation had been blown out of proportion and that the GP contacting Stella was a power play to exercise his authority over the hospital. I give Stella a brief account of the Mike situation and say we will act positively but assertively to ensure good communication between the doctors and nurses yet without succumbing to domination. Stella looked at me intently. I suspect she was hovering with a dilemma. I sense she wanted to assert nursing but on the other hand she wanted the problem to be smoothed over and dealt with. I sense she suspected further difficulties if the GPs are not appeased. She stood and smiled. 'That's good. I fully support you.'

In response I said, 'If I can help you in any way in your new role I should be pleased to.'

'I am interested in your clinical supervision approach. Perhaps we can meet and talk more of that'.

She left. The sweat quickly went cold under my arms. Yet why did I feel such pressure? The next day at the hospital, Luke was as nice as pie. Leslie was most attentive. Old norms had been reasserted.

Four weeks later I heard Myrna, another primary nurse, criticise Leslie for his 'defensive nursing' – she meant his extensive notes on a patient's discharge. Leslie agreed he was being defensive. He looked at me. He knew that I knew he was doing this to prove to Luke he was competent. I wanted to liberate him from his own censor that pulled hard at him, that subordinated him to the GP. I needed him to realise his own power. Old norms and patterns of learnt relationships are not easily overthrown. Yet the norm had been breached. Tension was on the surface where it could be dealt with.

Leadership is creating the learning organisation where we can learn from mistakes without blame and shame. Although we have systems in place through clinical supervision and standards of care groups, the primary nurses often feel isolated. I must invest more time in supporting and challenging Leslie and the other primary nurses.

Situations like this are good because it shakes people out of any complacency. Leslie was careless. He felt punished like a naughty boy. Big daddy (Luke) had scolded him. Big mummy (me) had comforted him and made it better. I wanted to admonish Luke for his behaviour but yielded. Not a time for showdown following the Mike incident. Being collaborative, I invited the GPs to attend the standards group to write a new standard of care on discharge even though I knew they wouldn't attend. They had made their point. They had scored the points. Being transformational in the transactional world is not easy. I must persevere.

Sheila

Some months later, Sheila knocked on my office door. I had deliberately closed it so she must knock – a power play playing the old hierarchical game.

I had summoned her to see me before she went home after her night duty. I am concerned about her comments undermining nursing practice. She was nervous, being summoned to speak with 'matron'. I invited her to sit down and tell me how she felt about nursing at the hospital. She confessed her yearning for the days of the old-style matrons when everyone knew where they stood. She liked order. She had never agreed with the previous changes and now it's happening again. We agreed that patient care was paramount, we just disagreed as to how we went about it. I invited her critical voice to be involved rather than as a separate harping voice that demeaned the hospital in the local community – a palpable threat to my own voice. She apologised. I was pleased she took responsibility for her actions. I smiled and thanked her. She said, 'I will retire soon so it won't make too much difference to me.' Typical of her to have the last word. I wondered if our conversation would make any difference. But that's not the point. The point was I confronted the hearsay, determined to be collaborative rather than competitive, investing in our relationship, investing in a better world based on compassion rather than hatred.

Making changes

Nelson writes: My employing PCT have stated that the development of one new initiative aimed at improving public health should be a key objective for each health visitor. As such, I am required to sign up to this as part of my individual performance and development review. This had seemed an impossible task a few months ago; now, I see it as a new opportunity for learning. The government white paper *Choosing health – making healthy choices easier* (Department of Health 2004b) sets new standards of public involvement in health care. *Choosing health* had its agenda set by the public following a period of unprecedented consultation – the paper calls this 'reconnecting with people's lives'. The core principles underpinning this new empowered public health approach are informed choice, personalisation and working together. This degree of public empowerment has long been a part of my personal vision for practice. I have experienced the value of allowing clients to set their own health agendas and witnessed the high levels of motivation for change in health-affecting behaviour that this brings. The real challenge lies in learning to extend this connection to whole communities and in finding new and innovative ways of listening to them and working with them to achieve health improvements.

Transformational leaders can be catalysts for change by expanding a holistic perspective, resulting in an empowered community able to direct their own health outcomes (Trofino 1995). One of the strategies I envisioned using to achieve this was a public consultation exercise. I felt I could commit to a regular session aimed at improving community health and while I was aware that I could decide what type of group to begin, this was clearly an opportunity to allow the public to set the agenda.

I contacted the health promotion team of my PCT for advice on the development of an 'open day' at a local surgery, hoping to provide an opportunity for listening to the community. I wanted to be as open as possible to their needs and then find the best way of meeting them. Crucially, this had to be best for them, not for me. A meeting between me, a colleague and two health promotion workers established a framework for the open day, and a date agreed.

I was conscious of the importance of leading this process effectively. I had very little previous experience in change leadership and recognised that changing how I lead change lies at the heart of effective leadership (Cope 2001). Cope (2001: 133/5) suggests using a change ladder to examine aspects of a proposed change and emphasises the need for honesty in evaluating the real values driving the change. The change ladder consists of five rungs to support the proposed change (Figure 5.7).

In my journal, I play with each rung of this change ladder. My motivation for change was a deep-seated belief in the potential for health visitors to make sustainable changes to health in the community. Encouragingly, Cope believes that at this level, change has the opportunity to be meaningful and effective.

Effective leadership is about effective communication. One model I find most helpful to help frame and reflect on leadership communication is Cope's styles of change leadership (2001) using a change matrix to establish the degree of visibility and planning (Figure 5.8). Exploring this matrix prompted a reflection of my change style. Cope argues that there are useful aspects in each style and that by using the emergent change matrix, a hybrid of all four change styles, a flexible and holistic style can develop. He writes (2001: 140), 'While your natural style and preferred change style might have

• The first rung is concerned with resources or assets.
• The second rung is concerned with a plan for change, what he describes as a blueprint.
• The third rung is concerned with the capability of staff to perform the envisaged change.
• The fourth rung is concerned with commitment or motivation for change – 'do we want this change?'
• The fifth and top rung is concerned with meaning and values.

Figure 5.7 Change ladder (Cope 2001)

Accidental (low planning/ low visibility)	You have a clear understanding of where you want to go, but you don't have a clear process of how to get there. You're happy to leave events to fate on the basis that the environment is so dynamic that overt control will never work.
Backstage (high planning/low visibility)	You have a clear plan of the way that the change will be managed, but much of the action takes place in corridors or shadow areas.
Controlled (high planning/ high visibility)	You follow a planned and visible structure of change, which means making the assumption that you can predict and control your future according to a set of rules.
Debate (low planning/high visibility)	Here shift happens through power of dialogue. You're open about the change and talk to people about the transformation, but don't have a structured approach to how it might be delivered.

Figure 5.8 Change style matrix (Cope 2001)

served you well to date, to survive and prosper in a turbulent world you need to have as broad a range of styles in your personal toolkit as possible.'

I realised that my natural style is 'controlled', using a highly planned and visible structure of change, and not conducive to transformational leadership. I was aware that this style was at odds with the empowerment model I hoped to develop and could prevent me being, and appearing to be, open to new ideas and ways of working. I became mindful of my need to develop aspects of each of these styles, particularly more of the accidental style which I hoped would give me the freedom and creativity that this project required. This style is concerned with subtly shifting the conditions of practice so change can flourish almost unnoticed, as if tuning into the inherent order within apparent chaos. Cope (2001) suggests learning to love the turbulence of the accidental style – the very aspect that my planning is usually geared to eliminate. Once I had reviewed my attitude to change and my natural style, I became more mindful of my approach and aware that I had the ability to change my own ways of leading change. This was an important step in the process. I felt empowered by the insights of my reading.

In a transactional world the controlled style is always viewed as preferable because it enables prediction and control. Yet such approaches tend to be rationally focused and pay little attention to the fact that successful change requires attention to both driving and resisting forces. Perhaps this is why so much change fails.

I was aware that I was moving out of my 'comfort zone' into a new way of learning and working. My journal documents my resulting feelings of strength and energy:

> This feels like sailing in uncharted waters, for I have no blueprint or experience to use, so I have to rely on instinct and the strength of my commitment. I am excited and daunted in equal measure, and everyone else seems to think I am mad. Have just got 'sorted', and now I'm jumping in at the deep end again.

I looked for a model of change to provide a framework for the experience, conscious that any rigid model would not be conducive to the 'accidental style' I am hoping to learn to feel comfortable with. Burnes' framework (1990) that details nine elements that constitute a facilitative approach to leadership (Figure 5.9) proved helpful. Whilst other models I explored focused on change as a problem-solving event, Burnes emphasises vision as a catalyst for change. He emphasises the value of continuous improvement; that change is not a single episode but an ongoing process of evaluation and re-evaluation. This idea fits well with the type of change I was planning, driven by vision and necessitating involvement and commitment from others for its success. I prefer to consider myself a leader rather than a manager of change but found the framework a helpful guide. I internalised the elements as a mental checklist to use as a reflective framework. Its emphasis on encouraging communication and dialogue, using regular feedback and progress reporting, was particularly useful and served as a timely reminder that this was a team effort.

The group agreed on two activities to facilitate the consultation process, a 'bull's eye' and a 'wishing tree'. The bull's eye used Velcro-backed cards around a large target stuck on a wall. Visitors will be encouraged to think of uses for the new room – things that they would use to help them achieve their own health objectives. The wishing tree is less specific – a large Xmas tree with stars that can be written on to decorate the tree with. These are for wishes for the community and can be for anything at all linked to improving health.

I consciously adopted a more relaxed style than I am used to, although everyone involved in the project is aware that I am the driving force. I am deliberately not chairing meetings, and no minutes are taken. Yet the 'accidental style' of Cope (2001) is proving difficult to sustain; people need more direction and perhaps want me to be more visible. So I consciously shift to the 'debate' style. This works well. My visibility motivates people. Decisions

• Creating a vision: mission, values outcomes, values conditions and midpoint goals
• Developing strategies: linked to vision, long-term considerations and present necessities
• Creating the conditions for successful change: raise awareness of the pressures for change, regular feedback, publicise successful change, understand people's fears and concerns, encourage communication and involve those affected
• Creating the right culture: encourage flexibility, autonomy and group working.
• Assessing the need for and type of change: identify the trigger, the remit, the assessment team, clarify the opportunity, investigate alternatives, give feedback and present recommendations and decisions
• Planning and implementing change: establish teams, activity planning, commitment planning, management structures, conduct post-audit and commence training
• Involvement: inform those affected, progress reporting, two-way communication and actual involvement via representation
• Sustaining the momentum: provide resources for change, give support to the change agents, develop new competencies and skills and reinforce desired behaviour
• Continuous improvement: encourage dialogue and examine work practices

Figure 5.9 Nine elements that constitute a facilitative approach to manage change (Burnes 1990)

are all reached by consensus. The 'debate' style works yet I am aware that not all change projects would be so simple. I had invited those involved because I knew that they were sympathetic to my vision of empowerment. My insight is that effective leaders appreciate different styles and can move easily between them in response to shifting conditions. My insight is that the leader needs to be mindful of which style she is using whilst always moving towards a debate style.

I am keen to emphasise a social model of health rather than a medical model and find no resistance to this concept at all except for one manager who expressed a tentative concern that I could be raising unrealistic expectations in the community by encouraging such free thinking. This was an important issue, and one that we addressed at the following and final meeting before the event.

I had originally considered a questionnaire but wanted to avoid pre-empting and limiting responses by the questions asked. I can see the value in these fun, visual and immediate strategies to facilitate real 'blue-sky thinking'.

The group all agree, however, that the whole ethos of the exercise is to encourage as broad a range of views as possible. While it is unethical to raise false hope, it is important to listen to the community without prejudice. We decide to make clear in our discussions on the day that there are no promises to deliver everything wished for, and this was when the title 'wishing tree' was coined (because as everyone knows, wishes don't always come true).

It was around this point, about a week before 'the day', when I realised that while much of my energy had been focused on planning this single event, the actual process of change and learning was already happening. Lewin's basic change model of unfreezing, changing and refreezing, which had initially seemed so unappealing and simplistic, began to make absolute sense (Lewin, cited in Schein 1999). I felt that I had been released from a frozen state of traditional practice to a more open state of heightened awareness, with motivation as a driving force.

Lewin (1935) suggested that the stability of human behaviour is an uneasy equilibrium of driving and restraining forces, and that increasing the driving force often results in an equally strong opposing reaction to counterbalance it. This force field analysis leads to the understanding that moving the equilibrium could be best achieved by removing the restraining forces, allowing the driving force naturally present to dominate.

My reprioritising and repatterning of care (Wuest 1998) had clearly removed a restraining force, allowing the driving force – my vision of an empowered community – to flourish. Without a vision for practice, others may not have the same driving force to promote change. Indeed, removing a restraining force to allow change could allow another restrainer – fear of change – to dominate.

This insight prompted me to offer to share my experience at the three-monthly meeting of all health visiting teams in my PCT. By hearing of my learning about change and my experiences, I hoped other teams may be less threatened by change and prepared to consider their own initiatives. Many expressed negative comments about trying anything new, and although I felt disappointed initially, it did serve to illustrate how much my leadership skills had developed.

Ottaway (1976) defines norms as the unwritten rules assumed by all. Gradually – and I recognise that this is a slow process, the drip-drip effect – a new cultural norm can be created, of community empowerment and partnership working.

The open day itself did not prove the enormous success I had hoped for – numbers attending were small, not helped by a thunderstorm raging the whole afternoon. Those who did attend nevertheless proved to be excellent at articulating their needs, with just a little encouragement.

A wide range of ideas were generated, and we are now working to provide a healthy walks scheme for women, first aid courses held in the village and a register of local community facilities. Some ideas were raised that were not within a health visiting remit but were important to acknowledge – letters to the local MP, parish council and county council have been sent on issues as diverse as street lighting, lack of play facilities for children on a large housing association new-build development, an overcrowded lower school and provision of poop bins for dog walkers.

It is difficult to be sure that I am effectively evaluating an event like the open day, for there are no criteria with which to measure success. It is even harder to evaluate a change such as client empowerment, particularly as I feel it is not my place to evaluate it, for in the spirit of empowerment, it should be the clients who evaluate it.

While I found Lewin's basic model of unfreezing, changing and refreezing led to some important insights, I now feel that I do not wish my changed approach to practice to be refrozen, for this implies repeating a similar process for every change. I prefer to think of my practice as remaining fluid, not refreezing at all, but able to adapt its shape according to need. Trofino (1995) cites Gaebler and Osbourne (1992) describing a new type of entrepreneurial public organisation that differs from traditional bureaucratic models in that it steers more than it rows. My vision is to neither steer nor row, but in terms of community empowerment, merely to provide the boat. Nevertheless, this change in practice requires strong navigational skills to steer health visiting practice into uncharted waters.

An important aspect of transformational leadership is the ability to test new ways of doing old things (Sofarelli and Brown 1998). I feel my commitment to making changes here demonstrates my emerging skills as a transformational leader, not afraid to make mistakes and to take risks in the pursuit of effective clinical public health practice.

Conclusion

Leadership is the vital ingredient for driving forward professional nursing practice and organisational development towards effective care. Some insights:

- The significance of vision as a prelude for all action, to act in tune with values, and that failure to adhere to this was a failure of integrity that undermined self-esteem.

- Knowing and managing my emotional tension when faced with difficult situations, notably a fear of sanction from those with greater positional power, had been and remained a powerful socialising force. Coming to understand this was one thing; shifting it was quite another. I call this poise.
- The effective leader must always intend a consistent collaborative style of managing conflict. I say 'intend' because the organisational culture mitigates against a collaborative style, infused as it is with issues of agenda, authority and emotional tension.
- The power of expertise – that could not be ignored because of my community hospital experience in Dorset.
- That influence was powerful when linked to positional power because positional power is the power people know and respond to. It is the balancing act of de-emphasising positional power and emphasising influential power.
- That to win hearts and minds the leader must be consistent, no matter what, that I had to walk the talk so to speak and invest in others to take responsibility and grow. Yet within the transactional organisation, it is not easy to relax one's grip on positional power as necessary to enable others to take responsibility and grow.

No doubt there are many more significant points of realisation. I realised now, with hindsight, how guidance would have been of great benefit and that leadership always needs mentoring because being submerged in the transactional culture it is not easy to rise above it and see beyond it to view things differently and realise true leadership.

Reflection

- How might you, as a leader, approach a potential change project?
- Identify potential driving and resisting forces using Lewin's force field analysis.
- How would you rate the staff you work with along Senge's commitment–apathy scale? As a leader can you shift people towards commitment?

Notes

1. www.brainyquotes.com
2. See also Chapter 4.

6 'No One Said This Would Be Easy'

Introduction

Leaders persist in hard times (Schuster 1994). Put another way, resilience is a vital attribute of leadership.

Resilience – '(of a person) able to recover quickly from difficult conditions' (Chambers 2005: 875). The meaning of resilience of an object is 'able to recoil or spring back into shape after bending, stretching or being compressed'. The transactional culture applies such pressure that people lose their ability to spring back. Under this pressure they are reshaped to conform with the organisation's shape. Only then is the pressure eased.

Okri (1997: 132) writes optimistically: 'Whatever resilience has kept wounded people and devastated nations here, alive, can be transfigured to make them strong, confident and serene. They have to question everything, in order to rebuild for their future. They have to re-dream the world. Freedom is the beginning of the greatest possibilities of the human genius. It is not the goal.'

Okri suggests that the energy of resilience can be transformed into a creative energy to rebuild people's future as leaders. In her narrative, Pia's quest is to break free from the shackles of oppressive transactional relationships in order to become a leader. When Pia shared her stories in the community of inquiry, other leaders shared similar stories. Resilience becomes a collective. In some ways Pia's narrative is remarkable in that people should face such oppression in their lives from others allegedly committed to health care. Perhaps 'committed' is the wrong word. Commitment becomes sublimated into tyranny within the transactional intent to control. As such, I subtitled the book 'Freedom to Lead'. Pia, like Martha (Chapter 2), was influenced by Schuster's characteristics of transformational leadership to mark her leadership emergence.[1]

Pia writes: For almost 30 years I have worked in the NHS; the last twenty-five as a practising midwife. I have been with my present NHS trust for 18 years in a variety of roles. Twelve years as a labour ward sister on permanent night duty had left me exhausted. A large part of me wanted to leave midwifery altogether. However, an opportunity appeared; I applied for and achieved a post in the antenatal/gynaecology clinic. I downgraded and reduced my hours. Colleagues expressed surprise and disbelief. Although the work was mundane and boring, the social hours were adequate compensation. The change of scene re-energised me and I decided to complete an academic module – the supervisor of midwives course. Later I successfully applied for the newly created practice development post in midwifery. My role was to support and guide the professional development of the midwives to enhance their practice.

When I commenced my leadership journey I had no vision of leadership. In fact I struggled to see beyond – 'what I do'. As Cope (2001: 49) states, 'true personal leadership must come from the inner strength of who I am rather than what I do'. Reflecting on these words I realised how I have always avoided looking at myself. I quickly realised I had a low self-regard despite my outward aura of confidence. Underneath my skin, if I am honest, I know I wear a mask. I am anxious about getting everything right, doing the right thing – a perfectionist. I know this is due in part to my upbringing. It was structured and constraining. Freethinking and questioning was not encouraged. This attitude characterised my education and my nursing and midwifery training. Realising my low self-regard was significant, I wanted to hide, but I knew that to become a leader I had to be *authentic,* to pull away the masks and face up to my real self and live the words of Johns (2004a: 139). 'In enabling the growth of self, the self needs to be honoured and valued. If we are unable to honour ourselves then we will be unable to honour those with whom we work, either our patients or our colleagues.'

Blowing the whistle

A year ago I 'blew the whistle' on my manager. Her planned falsification of training records in support of our directorate's insurance assessment would have implicated myself and other colleagues and potentially been extremely damaging to our organisation. In addition, my own professional accountability would have been completely undermined. By informing me of what she planned to do meant that I was implicated. However, I knew that exposing her professional neglect would mean considerable personal risk to myself, and indeed that proved to be the case. Although there was never any doubt in my mind that it was ethically the right thing to do, it took courage. Leadership *is* moral (Bass 1985, Cassidy and Koroll 1994).

I do not regret my actions although the consequences have left me bruised and exhausted. It was not a comfortable place to be. I couldn't move on. Each time the scab began to heal some small issue with her would trigger it off, and I would pick at it and make it bleed again. Although difficult and painful, I recognised through reflection, that *caring for self* is a skill I needed to learn.

Johns (2013) identifies that it may be difficult for the practitioner to focus on self, especially if the practitioner is well defended from looking in. My history goes against me; I am well defended against 'looking in'. I had to learn to step out of my skin and assert myself as a leader. Thus began a process of unlearning – coming to appreciate and letting go of old ways of doing things and managing self that were not congruent with my vision of self as a transformational leader.

However, leadership as an idea is one thing, and being a leader is quite another. I could feel the tension between expectations of myself to become a leader and expectations from others within the organisation to know my place within the normal pattern of transactional relationships.

Thus eventually, and I think *courageously,* I made a decision to initiate a meeting with my manager, Jane, to attempt to resolve the situation and draw a line under past events. Jane has not been my manager for very long. I was used to being managed quite loosely. Now it's different. Does Jane want to rein me in order to prove herself a good manager? Or is she simply anxious and controlling? Previously, *knowing my place,* I would not have initiated this meeting. I would have put up with it.

For me this meeting was to be what Cope (2001: 54) describes as a landmark – 'something that gives you a stake in the ground and a basis on which to make a decision. The ability to find a reference point in times of turmoil and confusion is an essential part of any leadership process.'

The meeting was planned for the afternoon. I felt tense all morning. Keeping my head down, in my office, I dreaded bumping into her in the corridor. My anxiety bit deep, but I felt prepared and in control. I had initiated the meeting. This was my choice. I felt empowered and strengthened by the fact that Jane had agreed to it. For months we have adopted this polite professional front. We had managed to get by.

We met. Deliberately I sat beside her rather than opposite. I realised immediately that she wanted to take control of the meeting. I let her take the lead. Let her speak. It was a conscious decision – it allowed me space to observe. In front of her was a list she had written. She went down it, methodically ticking things off as she went. It reminded me of a schoolteacher at registration. I focused hard on not feeling like a schoolgirl. I was not going to let myself be put in my place anymore. Jane identified how I constantly challenged her and how I was aggressive and always working to my own agenda. Rambling on and on. I tried to let the words wash over me, not to let them hurt me. But they did.

When she had finished I quietly and deliberately laid my cards on the table. I told her I didn't trust her. I had trusted her in the past, although now, I suspect our relationship had only ever been based on thin trust. I recall how she looked – surprised at my *honesty*. I felt secure as I negotiated with her a way to rebuild trust between us. A journal entry shows the depth of my feelings:

> I said to her that this was a going to be a big thing for me because if that trust proves to be misplaced then I sense the damage to myself and the organisation will be irreparable. I told her that I didn't do this lightly but that I have little energy left to fight (it really has felt like a battle) and that we need to come together and find some common ground to start again.

The meeting ended with our mutual agreement to put this whole episode behind us, to start afresh and move on. Bizarrely she asked for a hug. I was surprised and uncomfortable. I felt I couldn't refuse. Here was this powerful person showing a vulnerable childlike side. I hated it. I certainly didn't want to hug her. She wept, and I wept. It was awful. In the moment I felt no release, only discomfort. Yet the moment seemed powerful and somehow significant. I was exhausted, yet I felt stronger and more confident as a consequence. My self-regard up a notch!

That evening I wrote in my journal:

> I hope at last that this is a new start with Jane now. Today has been one of the most difficult and painful days for me personally within my whole career. I hated weeping and loss of control. Perhaps it did her good to see me cry? Cynical? We agreed to start afresh, draw a line and work professionally. I know that there is risk here, but it is a gamble I am prepared to take. This is my choice and I choose to move on leaving this behind.

The journal entry is positive. Everything is fine, all sorted. Yet I was kidding myself. I felt a deep sense of unease. How did Jane feel? Perhaps like me, she was trying to show a polished and professional front to the world, but underneath the surface she was brittle. However, it was to be a rare moment of her revealing herself to me. In the months ahead I was to forget all about her vulnerabilities as I became engulfed by my own.

Sharing the experience in the leadership group was affirming and insightful, despite feeling nervous of revealing myself and of opening my defences for scrutiny. Being in the group I felt accepted for who I was. I felt supported. I affirmed I would no longer avoid conflict with Jane – realising that avoiding conflict was my normal mode of operation. I felt as if I have stepped out of a dark corner and become visible, opening the possibility for a more collaborative type of relationship with Jane. I remind myself that in leading myself, I put myself in a better position to lead the midwives.

Time passed. I met regularly with Jane to update her on progress of work. I sensed we were now working quite well together, although occasional comments and gibes from her didn't go unnoticed. Perhaps I was naive to ignore them. Perhaps I was overly anxious to tick the box and think that the conflict within our relationship had been resolved. I was working so hard at trying to be transformational and was blindly confident. I didn't appreciate how soft the soil was that my leadership house was built on.

Back to the beginning

I journal:

> Today has been awful. Out of the blue a run-in with Jane. I had a catch-up session with her regarding some work and she accused me of being aggressive and always challenging her. Not again! I felt so upset; I thought that we had been getting along okay. Apparently yesterday I said that I didn't want to do a specific piece of work. I denied it but she very firmly said, 'Yes, you did say that.' The frustrating thing is I was only suggesting another way of looking at this work to involve other directorates. She twists my words to suit herself. Like a child I said, 'Well, I hope I am doing a good job.' She replied, 'Yes, you are. I would have told you if you hadn't. You have outgrown this job and you need to be careful that the aggression doesn't take you over.' This happened to me in another unit and I was labelled a troublemaker. Where did this come from?

I thought our relationship was going well. How mistaken I was! I remember the distorted look on her face as she waved her pen at me. I felt frightened that it was going to start again. The trust thinned between us, cracking. How easily I slip into the role of a hurt child!

I journal:

> Why does Jane make me feel like a hurt and rebellious child? Jane had become the critical parent. I know rationally that my interactions with Jane should be as an adult.

I tried to manage my anxiety by asking 'I hope I am doing my job properly' I was defensive, fearful of punishment, attempting to take back some control, but also childlike looking for praise and reassurance. Due to our respective anxieties, we are in adult–child regression – the classic transactional pattern.

I write fine words and think fine thoughts but in reality I recognise that I have not yet dealt with the internal conflict within myself that has, over such a long time, become internalised as self-depreciation and a habit of playing the 'victim'. Johns (2013) notes that the natural tendency to reflect is to defend self against anxiety rather than use this energy as a positive learning opportunity. How true this is for me! Early on in my journal writing I identified that most of my writing was indeed negative. I even developed a basic marker system that at the end of each entry I drew a happy or sad face. There were few happy faces.

I journal:

> It was liberating to be able to share this experience within my guided reflec-
> tion group. It guided me to see where Jane was coming from and the way
> her anxiety is typically transactional and transmitted down the hierarchy.

Entangled within the system I just hadn't seen this perspective. My insights are too superficial to shift my practice, although the contradiction feels stronger. I think I am acting like an adult but I still behave like a child. This makes me miserable. I need to channel my negative feelings of anger and despair into positive action in tune with my leadership values. I wonder if I am more comfortable being the oppressed victim even though it clearly makes me unhappy. These are deep questions to answer. Jane's warning about being labelled a potential troublemaker initially scared me. I didn't want to be labelled a troublemaker! Yet was that really going to be the case? I can't be a leader if I live in fear – the impact of coercive power (French and Raven 1968).[2]

Yet what am I afraid of? There is always a fear of being 'told off' but in reality what can they do to me? Again and again it goes back to the very centre of the person that I am – back to my childhood, back to my training, always trying to avoid being 'told off'. The leadership group helped me to see that I was in a stronger position with Jane than I seemed to think. In reality her power is brittle. It is my challenging that she sees as aggressive behaviour. In challenging her I reinforce her need to cling onto an outdated culture of hierarchical control. Essentially transactional in her approach she sees herself very much as my boss.

Holding to my leadership vision, I must persevere and push through fear. I sense a deeper understanding of the importance of being assertive and developing a genuine collaborative style in my work relationships, no matter where the other person is positioned in the transactional hierarchy.

Yet the conflict goes on.

I was sitting at my computer catching up with my emails – some precious space between teaching on the study day I am facilitating. The day is going smoothly. Clare comes bustling in. She says, 'I want to see you today instead of next week. Can you come around now?'

This is a meeting I had set up a few weeks ago before she went off for a month's study leave. There has been so much reorganisation within our directorate. Rumour is rife and I wanted to clarify my position and role within the organisation. I had heard that Clare is to become my manager again. Jane had told me that a significant number of projects would now be coming my way. I was anxious about this. I felt disempowered about not having a voice about my work and change of manager. After my experience with Jane I didn't want this change. I was pleased that I had taken the initiative to organise the meeting. Now I feel irritated, wrong footed by Clare bringing it forward.

Clare is not in the office at the appointed time. Several times I return to no avail as I juggled her demand around my own commitments. I feel uneasy. I try to organise my thoughts on how to manage myself within this meeting, telling myself, 'You've thought about it for long enough. Just go in there and keep it adult–adult. Be honest and try and communicate effectively. You know you are a good communicator so what's the problem?'

Eventually she's there. She looks tense, preoccupied. Even before I sit down I sense this was not going to go well. I glance at the photos on the desk of her children and husband. I take comfort from them. I try to relax, sit back on the chair, open my body and open my mind. I try to smile and look happy and positive like the photos on the desk, but I can't. Off she goes. She speaks at length about how she is planning to move things forward and how things need changing. I sit and listen. She acknowledges herself that she is rambling and garbled. Unconsciously I doodle on the wooden arm of the chair. So soon into the meeting I am feeling like a child. This is supposed to be my meeting but she clearly has her own agenda and I let her take over.

The phone rings and she tells me to leave the room whilst she takes the call. Ten minutes of sitting outside her office like a little girl waiting to go back in again, still unable to manage my anxiety, I think, *I am not a priority here.* If that had been me I would have excused myself and said I was in a meeting and would call them back. I would focus on the person I was with. I always try to demonstrate that *I have people's interests at heart* (Schuster 1994).

131

Back in her office. I deliberately avoid looking at the happy photos. At last my turn to speak. I speak of why I had asked for a meeting, revealing my concern about the significant increase in my workload and my disquiet at the change of line manager, not being consulted in this decision, and that I was no longer clear about my place in the organisation. I suggest that the lack of consultation and openness in her approach is having a detrimental effect on the team as well as me. Despite her signals, I persist in getting my points across. I sense I'm beginning to turn the meeting around.

She says how disappointed she is at my reaction. She had expected me to see it as an opportunity. I should accept that although we were a small team, I should understand that there are tiers and that I am reacting to the ripples of change. My attempt to persist and show courage came to an end. I didn't even try and engage further with her. I didn't have the energy. What would be the point? She is so transactional. I let her words go in, like a knife – stab, stab. Each stroke opening my old wound. I leave feeling extremely despondent.

I journal:

> This has been such an awful day! Leadership? I feel like giving it all up. I really tried to challenge and demonstrate transformational leadership to self and others today – what a joke! But I am not laughing as I write; I'm weeping – tears of frustration, exhaustion and hopelessness. Just when I think I am moving forward on this journey up the mountain another boulder looms in front of me. So what is the learning? Don't bother to challenge because the personal cost is too painful? Yet it is such a huge dilemma because I sense I am too far down the road. Not to challenge for me now is an even greater cost – no progress, no moving forward. Despite this setback I choose not to take that option. I am not going to let this knock me back.

Despite my lamentation, my reflection affirms I will persevere in my leadership quest. I wonder, did I act for the best in going ahead with the meeting? Perhaps when Clare said 'I want to see you today', it became her meeting. Perhaps I could have asked 'Why the need now?' and then made a decision whether to comply. I say 'comply' because it felt like a demand. Either way, it felt like a no-win situation.

I try to see Clare's perspective; I sense she is stressed because of a directorate issue I know she is trying to resolve and other loose ends too, before going on a month's study leave. Her own position has recently been reviewed and eroded and she feels vulnerable. Perhaps she wanted to ensure that I didn't miss the opportunity to meet with her. Perhaps, as my manager, she expects to set the agenda for our meeting. I recognise this as a pattern with both Jane and Clare. My autonomy was being squashed and I could not assert it. I had disappointed her. Again the naughty girl reminded of her place. Where is respect? Perhaps that hurts most.

As head of midwifery, Clare uses authoritative power to demand compliance with her agenda, always with a threat of sanction if I resist and potential reward if I comply. It is the corrosive nature of transactional power in stark contrast with the transformational power I seek to cultivate within my patterns of relationship.

I journal:

> Tradition, authority and embodiment are huge barriers for me to change myself.[3] I feel my oppression is deeply embodied.

I allude to Fay's notion that power, tradition and embodiment are barriers to rational change (Fay 1987). Put another way I have embodied my own subordination through transactional relationships that have reinforced my subordination. Such relationships are difficult to shift because they are normal and part of the transactional culture. In other words it is normal despite my unease. Now that I can see this pattern my unease and frustration grow. But I do have power! I do not have to be a victim of oppression! I can confront tradition by being mindful of myself within every interaction.

Sharing this experience with the leadership group, I am guided to draw a distinction between front and back foot thinking.[4] Being caught on the back foot means we are always dancing to another's tune whereas being on the front foot enables me to lead the dance. I always seem to be caught on the back foot with my managers. Can I revision being on the front foot where I can give Clare back her oppression? The thought liberates me but walking the talk is another thing.

At one point during the leadership group, in response to my protestations about trying to change, I was taunted: 'You will just get back into your box like a good little girl because that's what's expected of you.' His words hit home, hit a nerve. Briefly, I took them personally but I see now of course that is not how they were meant.

I journal:

> I have to see emotional tension for what it is, not to drown in it, but convert it into creative tension.

Someone in the group said, 'You've rattled her cage' – words that help offset my feeling of disempowerment and failure. Yes, I did rattle her cage, and a year ago I would certainly not have contemplated doing that. But I mustn't see that as compensation. I am not a victim. I must not take things so personally. Stop living in false fear (Beck 1997: 61).

I take comfort in the words of Okri (1997: 52): 'There are many ways to die and not all of them have to do with the extinction of life. Many of them have to do with living; living without asking questions; living in the cave of your own prejudices and living the life imposed on you.'

I am not willing to die in my cave! This experience was a true moment of understanding. Out of the carnage I felt a connection to a new leadership self.

Moving forward

A few weeks later. Five o'clock on a Friday night. I go to the delivery suite to hand over the unit bleep. I have spent a significant part of the day sorting out staffing issues for the weekend. Now I'm tired and glad to be going home. It's quiet with only one woman who has delivered. Several midwives and a student sit around the desk chatting. I wonder why I hadn't got the G grade to sort out the staffing issues to take the pressure of myself. That would have been a more transformational way to lead! Old habits are hard to shift.

The phone rings. It is the day assessment unit. It closes at five o'clock. Faith, the G grade who took the call, willingly agrees to accept a patient from them. At this point Cathy (another G grade) and Lisa (F grade) complain loudly. Cathy says, 'Every day from half four they start shipping patients over here. I'm sick of the way they go home early and dump on us.'

> I ask Cathy, 'Have you worked on the day assessment unit?'
> She replies, 'No, but I don't need to I know what they are like.'
> Lisa chips in, 'Well, I've worked there, and it's dead easy.'

The student looks on, bemused. I've heard enough. We have had much discussion in recent months within our senior management team around what can only be described as an increasingly disrespectful culture within the unit. Some of this lack of respect is directed to colleagues and sometimes towards patients during handover time, perpetuated by a small clique of midwives. These two are part of that clique.

It is time to demonstrate my leadership. I speak to them both deliberately and publicly suggesting that they should be more circumspect about the way they speak about their colleagues. I say that my office is next door to the day assessment unit and as such I'm aware of how hard they work. I hear it and see it. Deathly silence. They look uncomfortable. Lisa turns away, flushed and embarrassed. Not a sound. They are surprised. This is unusual behaviour for me, not what they would expect. I have an appointment with Lisa booked for the following week for her annual supervisory review. As I turn and walk away I wonder if she will cancel and perhaps request a change of supervisor.

I journal:

> I really feel that I have had a positive experience today. It was a big step forward for me. It was an opportunity to demonstrate leadership. Instead of shying away from it and wishing I had done something about it afterwards I just took the risk and said something. I have a real sense that it was the right thing to do. There was a student sitting listening as well as Faith, who had readily accepted the patient. It is really important that if I am to be credible with self and others I need to show that – almost as a role model. At the end of the day we are all supposed to be here for the patient. Where was she in all of this? I hope/think my behaviour gave them all something to think about. This certainly is a way of living life!

I remind myself that transformational leaders *evince a concern for the whole – reflected in a passionate and ethical voice being heard when necessary*[5]. In the past, I would not have had the courage to speak out like this. I am beginning to overcome the need to be liked in order to be true to the vision of 'being with woman'. Culture shock. *My behaviour is beginning to align with my words.*[6]

However, my response was the 'critical parent' in response to my anger. Perhaps I could have confronted them in a more 'adult' way? And yet, on reflection, it felt appropriate to act parentally when the 'children' are so irresponsible. Perhaps only then do they feel the issue.

I journal:

> Perhaps an edge of positional and even coercive power[7] is handy to keep up the sleeve because it is the language they understand.

I need to be mindful of my 'critical parent' response to my anxiety. I really did need to feel powerful to take the action I took. But does that legitimise my approach? I am mindful that this experience is not with people whom I deem to have power over me. If leadership is about doing the right thing then my use of positional power was problematic. Leaders should make things happen. I sense that I need to use my power in a positive way to tackle the issue and role model in ways that reinforce responsibility rather than as the critical parent.

Positive progress

As a supervisor of midwives, one of my role responsibilities is to meet annually with my supervisees to ensure that they are fulfilling their registration requirements. Lisa is one of my supervisees and our meeting was booked for the week following the previous experience. I was anticipating with some discomfort that Lisa may raise some issues.

I journal:

> A very surprising supervisory meeting with Lisa today. We got to the end of the meeting, which was uneventful. Part of me was disappointed that she hadn't mentioned last week. I wanted to follow it through so I gave her an opening right at the end. 'Is there anything else you want to discuss?' She seemed to take a breath and said there was. I thought – oh, here it comes. But it was not what I expected. She talked about the inequality of allocation of patients on the delivery suite by some of the G grades. How she understood that they needed to be relatively free as they were in charge but that often she would be allocated two or three patients whilst they had none. If one of hers was high risk it was unsafe. Lisa also highlighted that although Cathy was her friend she was often the culprit. She was struggling to manage it and wanted guidance as to how to resolve it.

This was not what I expected. I was pleased Lisa could trust me to share her concern, despite the previous week's experience. Perhaps she realised I did have her best interests at heart. Leadership creates unexpected possibilities. My own journey of learning is recognising and understanding what the 'real' issues are. So what were the real issues? The issues for both of us were different yet intertwined. I wanted to focus on and explore the attitude and culture within the unit with Lisa and her friends as part of the problem. Lisa on the other hand wanted support on how to best confront someone who she publicly acknowledges as her friend and whom she also aligns herself with in the clinical area. I do not see Lisa in a positive way, an attitude honed on her past behaviour. She is a young and competent midwife who tends to come to work, do the job and go home. It is difficult to engage her in other activities that would support her development and the unit as a whole. This attitude is the norm within the directorate.

I ask Lisa to reflect on her vision of her role as a midwife in our directorate.

She identifies:

- To Offer a high standard of care to mothers and babies
- To Maintain skills to achieve this
- To Work within the NMC (Nursing and Midwifery Council) rules and standards

Lisa does all those things and does them well but her vision does not take in the bigger picture. She only takes responsibility for herself and not the organisation; she is not seeing how Cathy's actions impact on the whole. If Cathy is behaving like this with her then it is safe to assume that she is the same with other midwives, many of whom are more junior than Lisa and, as a consequence, are less likely to speak out. Where is the patient in this situation? I suggested to Lisa that we put her personal vision within the wider framework and context of the organisation.

She identifies:

- Ensure a high standard of care for *all* clients
- Facilitate professional relationships at work
- Recognise that there is also responsibility as a professional to view the bigger picture

I challenge her with the contradiction between these values and the way she acts on the unit. She is surprised. By involving and engaging with Lisa in this way I offered her a sense of vision ownership – an invitation to realise this vision rather than adhere to unprofessional behaviour that disadvantages both colleagues and the women we purport to support through childbirth.

She is thoughtful. I have pulled her out of her crowd. How will she respond when back in the normal culture? My engagement with Lisa helped me realise Schuster's transformational leadership attribute: – '*Your natural tendency is to develop others to become engaged, deepen perspectives and be effective.*' The words *natural tendency* feel rather hopeful. Maybe in time, but just now I feel it is more a forced intention.

Confident development

This morning my shared and often noisy office was quiet and empty. I was glad of the peaceful space as it enabled steady progress through my work. A knock on my door. 'Could I have a quick word?' I want to say 'no'. I look up at Alice's face. It is strained and full of sadness. I give her my full presence. She speaks of her unhappiness around her relationship with Clare and her decision to deselect herself as a supervisor of midwives. I am sorry but not surprised. Alice used to be the manager of the postnatal ward but when Clare came into post she was hastily redeployed to a community post with little discussion. No one knew why, not even Alice. Clare has given Alice a hard time in the monthly supervisors' meetings and Alice struggles to fight back. Her attempts to challenge are constantly rebuffed by Clare. Yet Alice is a senior midwife and a most experienced supervisor. I sense her inner struggle and conflict. Her loss to the organisation, the midwives and women would be significant. What of her loss to self? We sit and talk. Alice *trusts me*; she values my opinion. *I genuinely want to help her resolve her problem.*

I guide her to tease out the two separate issues. One is the fact that she has long-standing personal/historical issues with Clare that have never been addressed. The second is that although Alice is committed to supervision, she finds the workload onerous and the regular on-call commitment a real problem. Alice is a single parent who wrestles to find balance between her genuine and heartfelt commitment both to work and family. Maybe she is using the excuse of her problems with Clare as a reason to give up her supervisory role that deep down she no longer feels able to commit to. Maybe she has been worn down to a point of burnout.

We conclude that she needs to speak with Clare and confront the issues. I share my own conflict story so Alice does not feel alone and tell her how transactional analysis has helped me realise the transactional pattern of communication between us. Alice acknowledges this and says our talk has helped her look at the conflict with Clare from a different perspective. She leaves, hopefully more positive. I close the door and resume my work.

I journal:

> Today has been a good day for leadership. I have a real sense that in learning to lead self I am beginning to surface understanding of how to lead others. I feel more confident that I will be able to deal with Clare much better myself in the future if another episode of conflict rears its head! Although the situation Alice shared with me today is sad, it only reinforces what I already know about the transactional culture/leadership in this directorate.

Kirkham (1999) recognised that when midwives reflect on their experiences of the culture within midwifery, similar descriptions emerge. Midwifery is seen as essentially a culture of women that emphasises, and internalises, the values of caring and commitment irrespective of personal sacrifice. This ethic of service, fundamental to midwifery as a caring profession largely composed of women, often appears to put great pressure on midwives. Thus the very nature of this ethic, and the respect accorded to those who uphold it, makes it exceedingly hard to challenge. This suggests that working within a culture of caring and self-sacrifice may not actually equip midwives with the skills to support and care for each other. To me this is such a painful contradiction – the need for support and the fact that the culture of midwifery neither acknowledges nor provides for that need. It is ironic that the major part of the midwife's clinical role is to support and guide child-bearing women in ways which increase their confidence and ability to cope. Yet many midwives' loyalty to their organisational culture prevents them from acknowledging themselves as deserving of similar support and care or seeing the potential for developing their professional confidence and coping skills. I cannot solve Alice's problems for her. That responsibility is hers. However, I am glad that I could support her.

I journal:

> It had been mutually empowering, reminding me that leadership is being in relationship with others – being with person, not doing things to people. Transformational leadership reflects the midwifery ethos of being with woman.

These sessions with Lisa and Alice affirm my leadership potential. Yet the experience with Alice reminds me of my own disempowerment with Clare. I can guide others to assert self rather than avoid but can I move this boulder for myself? I didn't have long to wait.

Back to the beginning again

I have a meeting with Clare planned later this afternoon. These are fortnightly 'catch-up' sessions where my ongoing work is reviewed. I do not look forward to them. They make me feel that I have to justify my existence. However, today, I feel positive, fuelled by my experience with Alice. I go to her office at the appointed time. The door is closed. I listen and hear voices. I don't want to interrupt so I go away yet already I'm stressed. Ten minutes later I return. Still engaged. I write a note, 'Please ring me when you are free', and tape it on the door. I am trying to take back some control. As I write it I hope the door won't open and catch me like a silly schoolgirl. The note looks pathetic. Why have I slipped back into this place so easily? Again I go back. So much for taking control and being assertive – why not wait until she rings? The note is still there. I hang about and then the door opens. She sees the note and screws it up. She says, 'Oh, right, our catch-up session. Why didn't you knock?'

I say, 'I didn't like to interrupt.' I feel in the wrong, slipping so easily into my child ego state. She says she has to leave in about three-quarters of an hour for a hair appointment so there is no time for my catch-up session. Instead she spent the time sorting out issues around three drug users who were currently patients within the unit. I chased around and found sets of notes for her. I sat there while she made phone calls and nodded and agreed with what she said. What a good girl I am! Social services, child protection, drug liaison all get to speak to the head of midwifery, but not me.

The clock moves on. I extend the doodle on the chair arm I had made before – it feels like an old friend. I am angry with myself and totally disengaged. Clare goes for her hair appointment and the meeting is rescheduled.

I journal:

> Another waste of time – catch-up session with Clare. I was all prepared and nothing! Again a deep pervading sense of feeling undervalued. I really recognise these days that her behaviour and leadership style is so transactional. It was not her role to chase after these people; it should be Val's (out-patient services manager). I would have thought she should have handed this over to Val. Maybe she likes the power of being in control of everything. What I should have done was follow through with the note and not go running back like a child. At least once I was embroiled in the non-meeting I should have disengaged myself from the situation and rearranged the meeting. How easy it is to look back after the event and see the sense. Not so easy at the time! I guess this is what reflection is all about. I need to be much more mindful within the unfolding moment, live it and breathe it. It still all just seems such a struggle I feel like I am walking through wet concrete.

Transactional analysis

Repeating patterns. Transactional analysis (TA) helps me view my patterns of relationship with Clare. I slide down the mountain every time into child mode, angry at my failure to assert my agenda and shed the sense of fear. Power and its consequences can be perceived through observing and analysing patterns of relationship between people made visible through reflection using TA. In TA theory, people communicate from their respective ego levels – child, adult and parent:

> P – The parent ego develops with particular types of responsibility relationships when others are dependent on them for whatever reason. Parent ego can be critical, tolerant or comforting.
> A – The adult ego represents the person who is able to reason and take responsibility for self.

C – The child ego seeks instant gratification and is irresponsible. Child ego can be rebellious, conforming or hurt child. The child grows up and develops the capacity for reason and responsibility for self. (Berne 1961, Stewart and Joines 1987).

In terms of being adults, the healthy pattern of communication is adult-adult. This is the transformational leader's norm and necessary pattern for dialogue. The leader is mindful of her own ego state and enabling the other to be in adult ego state. When ego levels are reciprocated, for example, adult–adult, parent–child, effective communication can take place. When the pattern is not reciprocated communication breaks down. When people become anxious for whatever reason, they perceive a threat to their ego. In response, they move subconsciously into script-learnt patterns of responding to their anxiety where they feel more comfortable. These scripts are either parent or child mode. Hence adults tend to move into parent script when faced with the threat of losing control and losing respect from others or self-respect. They move into child script when faced with the threat of persecution, rejection and being overwhelmed (Barber 1993). Transformational leaders are adept at being and staying in adult mode even when they are anxious. Anxiety is a trigger to be mindful of their response. When relationships within organisations are largely based on authoritative sources of power (Figure 5.3), it is inevitable that managers, like Clare, respond to the high level of organisational anxiety by moving into parental script in order to control the situation. The consequence is that the subordinate other person compensates by shifting into child script as a learnt response to authority's insidious threat of sanction. I know that Clare oscillates between critical and nurturing parents. At times she is a critical parent when things do not go smoothly, projecting her anxiety onto me and no doubt others, classified as naughty children. At other times she flips into a nurturing parent script when it's obvious I am hurt. Trying to stay in adult mode just seems to make Clare more parental as if I am a threat to her control. Then communication breaks down and we are in tatters. It seems easier to move into child ego state for the sake of peace. Yet, in doing so, I fail miserably as a leader. It is vexing.

My narrative proves that parent–child patterns do not foster growth, preoccupied as they are with managing anxiety. Clare laments that staff lack responsibility yet it is she who creates the situation whereby myself and others can't take responsibility. It is even deeper than that. I sense the whole organisation has embodied this parental culture. It is like a toxic current flowing through the transactional organisation influencing subordinate behaviour.

At the next leadership group I admit I am disillusioned. I say to myself, *It's okay to struggle. We learn to yield rather than persist and see self as a failure.*

141

Those words stay with me like a talisman. In the community I am asked to stand up and measure my self-regard – the top of my head is the maximum. I protest, mumbling on about differences between self-regard at home versus work. I don't want to reveal the truth. Gently I am pushed to respond. I am honest. What's the point otherwise? I touch below my knees. The guide tells me, in truth, what I already know – that Clare leaves me disempowered and disabled. Another member of the group observes that I always seem to 'do myself down'. I know that what they say is right. It is a behaviour that I have adopted for years almost wanting to seek reassurance and praise from others by offering a negative image of self. Forever the victim.

Roberts (2000) identifies that one of the major factors that keeps the oppressed from becoming empowered is poor self-regard and identity. With a flattened self-regard it is difficult for me to be assertive and demand respect. This has to stop. I need to change the way I live my professional life in order to develop a more positive identity. If I am unable to realise this then I will not be able to work towards changing the organisation that oppresses others as well as self. Surely if I hold onto my vision strongly enough then I will realise it.

Later that night I wrote a poem.

> It's okay to struggle
> At least I am travelling
> I wasn't sure I could even start the journey
> Yet I am well on my way
> Do I travel well?
> Sometimes
> I sense I make good progress
> Striding out
> Stepping over stones
> Walking around boulders
> Enjoying the view
> But then there it is
> Looming
> Shingle and scree
> Grey and unforgiving
> There is no way around
> I have to climb
> I want to climb
> On and up
> I am bold and confident
> I pause I begin to slide
> The stones scrape and cut

I feel the pain
I dig my heels in
I will not slide back
It's okay to struggle.
Yet find another way.

Yet find another way. I have to learn to think about my thinking so I don't keep scraping my knees.

I must *honestly* address my relationships with those who I deem to have power and authority over me. If not, I will never realise my leadership vision. I choose whether to continue picking at the scab of this old wound. I recognise that if I push and try too hard against the forces that restrain me I may not overcome them. Without doubt, becoming a leader ain't easy!

I journal:

> Clare is a 'paper tiger flapping in the breeze'. No substance. Our guide leads the group into a meditation to bring the self home; to remember our visions and touch our personal power. He reminds the group that leadership is a spiritual quest. A wave of stillness envelops me, easing my suffering. Remember the breath when anxiety rises.

Although battered and bruised I do feel more confident about where I am going. As I draw the threads of my experiences together I discern a pattern. It is a pattern I will now change and weave in a different way, starting with love and respect for myself. Boyd (1996: 52) writes of time spent observing a Native American leader, Rolling Thunder: 'I can tell you that understanding begins with love and respect. Such respect is not a feeling or an attitude only. It's a way of life. Such respect means that we never stop realizing and never forget to carry out our obligation to ourselves.'

Of all that I have learnt, this understanding of self is the most important and valuable learning of all. This is a deeply charged and emotional realisation for me. It is impossible to convey in words the profundity and intensity of it. I acknowledge that at last the heart dimension is truly in place and I know that I can move on.

Empowerment

The sun shines through the dusty windows as I walk down the corridor. Bright, busy, changing patterns on the floor. Spring is coming. A fresh start. I smile – it's how I feel. Confidently I knock on Clare's door, no anxiety. I am strengthened by the previous leadership group session. *I feel powerful.* As I sit down, I notice my doodle on the chair arm. It is fading, perhaps reflecting a fading away of the old me.

The meeting is completely different from the last one. I engage positively about several pieces of project work that I am moving forward. Clare listens. Amazingly, in attempting to address the negative culture within the unit, she intends to put together a one-year leadership programme for senior midwives. I know this reflects the discussions I have initiated within senior team meetings around culture and leadership. Within the moment, and perhaps cynically, I consider whether she ever reflected on her own style of leadership, and its significance and relevance as to why we were having this conversation. We have a constructive exchange around her proposal and she is keen for me to draft some of my own thoughts for discussion at the next senior team management meeting. I don't mind the pervading sense that this is all her idea. I don't mind that I'll be doing the groundwork. I am reminded of Schuster's words – *I do not have a prominent dark side of ego power.* In fact I feel quite excited. I leave her office for the first time feeling able to *celebrate the now.* Is this empowerment?

I went to the meeting on the front foot,[8] mindful of *projecting my power into the room.* Sharing my expert knowledge around leadership was extremely empowering. I felt huge freedom. The last group leadership session had helped move a huge boulder. I am finding my voice. Not loud, but strong. I can now take responsibility for myself. No longer the willing victim anxiously picking at my wound. A ripple of confidence surges through me. I sense I can become a transformational leader. I feel the sharp curve of acceleration.

Endings

When I first sat down to write this work, facing a blank computer screen, unsure of how to start, I wrote a poem. I have returned to it many times. It has supported me and helped me centre my thoughts. As I close this tale of my leadership journey so far I wonder, have I reached the top of my mountain? In truth I sense I have. Yet now there is compulsion and need to walk on to the next ridge and scale new heights. The journey goes on; it is the journey of my life.

> *My last mountain?*
> *It just seems too big a mountain*
> *I can't even see the top*
> *I know I have to reach the summit*
> *I want to*
> *Yet I can't seem to 'see' how.*

I have climbed so many mountains to get to the foothills of this one
How easy to forget the journey now it's almost ended
I want to stop for good
Set up camp and curl up in my tent
Warm, dry and safe ... happy?
But then I will never reach my journey's end
Does that matter?
In truth it probably only really matters to me
I know I have come too far to turn back
I must look for a way around this mountain
Climb on and up and not be scared of falling
Somewhere there is a path to take
Even though I know when I get to the top
See the view, breathe the air and bask in my success
That I will see another mountain.
For deep down I know this journey never ends.

Conclusion

Pia's narrative is a salutary tale of liberation which graphically illuminates the nature of transactional management. Perhaps Pia was unfortunate to be managed by such people. I do not think so, simply because such relationships are normal within the transactional culture. Her poem 'My Last Mountain?' is evocative of her journey in that she can rest a moment yet knowing her leadership quest continues. She says, 'I know I have come too far to turn back.' It is the moral nature of leadership that once realised it becomes immoral in any other way without compromising her integrity. Being mindful she creates space to see the transactional organisation for what it is. She is less entangled, more poised and more resilient. She persists.

Reflection

- Reflect on a series of conversations you have with different people. Plot the transactional analysis pattern. When you recognise you are not in adult–adult mode, ask yourself 'Why is that?' and 'What must I do to stay in adult–adult mode?'
- How persistent and resilient are you? Write some experiences that reveal these qualities in you. How can you become more resilient?
- Write your own resilient poem.

Notes

1. See Figure 2.1.
2. See Figure 5.3.
3. Here Pia alludes to Fay's notion that power, tradition and embodiment are barriers to rational change (Fay 1987).
4. See Figure 1.6.
5. Schuster (1994) leadership attribute.
6. See note 5.
7. Here, Pia is alluding to French and Raven's typology of leadership power; see Figure 5.2.
8. See Figure 1.6.

7 The Road to Oz

Introduction

Becoming a leader can be viewed as a process of self-deconstruction and reconstruction, identifying and pulling away redundant assumptions and behavioural patterns and replacing these with new assumptions and behavioural patterns congruent with a vibrant vision of leadership. In this process, contradictions between vision and reality are dissolved until leadership becomes a lived reality.

> Lisa writes: This is the story of my personal leadership journey I call 'The Road to Oz'. It is a journey that changed me forever. Consider: the tin man had no heart; the lion lacked courage; Dorothy lived in fantasyland; whilst the scarecrow had no stuffing. On the road they got lost, encountered cruelty, overcame barriers, yet they persevered. My journey was finding all these things for myself as metaphors for leadership.

At the beginning I was the intensive care unit's practice development nurse. Before that I had been one of the unit sisters. Halfway along the journey I became the modern matron. Shifting roles yet leadership is constant.

How can such journeys be meaningfully communicated when they are so complex? It wasn't a simple linear process of one step in front of the other. I felt as if I was battling against one half of myself who was reluctant to make the effort and resistant to change. To represent the first 18 months of my journey, I constructed a jigsaw to deconstruct my existing mental models that seemed to represent my current reality working within the transactional organisation. In the second ten-month part of my journey, I reconstructed the jigsaw based on a new set of mental models that represented my emerging reality as a transformational leader.

Like Dorothy, I started along the road as a young, naive leader. On my journey I experienced many situations and theories from which I gained insight into my way of being as a leader and person. I reflected on where I came from, the steps of learning I experienced and where I am at now on that never-ending journey. I came to view the story as parts of my leadership puzzle. As my journey unfolded, these pieces of puzzle began to take shape.

The first piece of the puzzle was appreciating my lack of reflective skills and getting a real vision of leadership. I was wrapped up and suffocating in ideas of leadership and my reflective skills were superficial to say the least! The literature was in my head, not in my heart. Leadership is about passion and I lacked it.

	Poor reflective skills (no insight into self)	Lacks vision of leadership

Developing reflective skills was not easy for me. I couldn't find a way to move beyond the superficial into deeper aspects. I knew I resisted reflection and this quest for self-understanding. With perseverance and constant encouragement within my community of inquiry I began to discover the power of stories and the truth they spoke to me as the author. My reflections literally become a window into my soul. I found revealing myself to myself difficult and uncomfortable. I tried to rationalise and hide from the truth, but in revealing to others in guided reflection, I was confronted with my reality. I had nowhere to hide. It was disturbing and yet astonishingly liberating as I came to trust myself and the group. I became real even if that sounds corny.

Pinar (1981: 184) writes, 'we write autobiography for ourselves, cultivating our capacity to see through outer forms'. As a private person this was not something I could easily do. If my autobiography were for my eyes only I could excel. My dilemma materialised when I realised others would hear or read it. However, the revelations have been worth the discomfort. I was slow to grasp the essence of it. There were, however, moments of dramatic revelation.

Alongside my reflections on my leadership (or rather my lack of leadership), I began exploring leadership literature challenged with constructing a vision of leadership. My head spun with ideas that were not heartfelt. They weren't my ideas and I struggled to understand them. However, I did feel I was at the beginning of something important. The group's insistent hand held me even as I baulked.

This was the start of my long, but exciting journey to my goal – the all-knowing Oz. When I found this elusive character I felt sure everything would become clear and miraculously my transformation would be complete. But I quickly found that being cognisant of theory means little or nothing and you have to live it. As Nigel Crisp said, 'what we do is more important than what we say'.[1] It took me a long time to really absorb this.

Without doubt I am a conflict avoider and the contradiction this posed for a budding transformational leader is the next piece of my puzzle. Evidently I am not alone. It seems that most nurses and nurse managers are conflict avoiders (Cavanagh 1991), perhaps reflecting the socialisation of nurses as subordinate within the health care system over time. Reviewing my journal it seems that every experience I reflected on was infused with a degree of conflict. Clearly, conflict was part of my everyday practice and how I respond to it as a leader is vital. I learnt that even a slight shift in conflict response towards a more mindful and collaborative approach sets in motion a positive spiral that gathers momentum, raising a head of steam.

Conflict avoider (no possibility of learning)	Poor reflective skills (no insight into self)	Lacks vision of leadership

Reviewing these situations of conflict, I can see they stemmed from people intent on imposing their different agendas, my own included! I recognised that if conflict is not dealt with expertly, using a collaborative style,[2] virtually all attributes of transformational leadership are compromised. I had to see conflict as a positive word, as an opportunity to learn. Without doubt, as Blake and Mouton noted way back in 1964, conflict can be positive and encourages creativity and change.

At its root conflict is about power and control and lack of shared vision, as if vision has become clouded in the busyness of doing. As for my vision of leadership, in truth I had not considered my position. Factually, the year-long RCN (Royal College of Nursing) leadership course and the LEO course taught me many things and were at times inspiring, but I had never stopped to think, *How does this apply to me? What sort of leader am I? Am I effective?*

As I began to construct my personal vision of leadership so I began to work with my colleagues to unravel a shared vision of practice, to find (recover?) meaning in our practice. How could I be a transformational leader without a vision for myself and for my organisation? We did have a vision on the unit yet no one knew who wrote it. It was an artifact comprised of fuzzy words that had no real meaning. And so I, we, began to polish it with vigour.

Fuzzy vision of practice		
Conflict avoider (no possibility of learning)	Poor reflective skills (no insight into self)	Lacks vision of leadership

Porter O'Grady (1992) found that managers are often selected on their ability to maintain the status quo. This idea resonated within me. It made me consider my position within the organisation – why did I think I had been chosen for my leadership role? Did the organisation expect me to maintain the status quo or be someone who would challenge and transform it? I was not sure. I felt my tension rise. My reflections forced me to admit that although I worked in an area of intense change, on a personal level I despised change. I prefer the status quo, keeping control, where I do not risk, experiment and learn as Schuster (my leadership guru) extorts me to as a transformational leader.[3] My desire to maintain the status quo thus became the fifth part of my puzzle. A gradual realisation of my mental models at my deepest level was emerging into consciousness, aspects of self that I had never explored before. I could not have imagined a leadership programme could be so personal. I had thought it would simply explore ideas to take away. It was more like a cookery-intensive than takeaways!

Likes status quo (likes to be in control)		
Fuzzy vision		
Conflict avoider (no possibility of learning)	Poor reflective skills (no insight into self)	Literature in my head not in my heart

I didn't know it at the time, but a line can be drawn here of my progress along the road to Oz as if I had reached a place of no return if I stepped further. Perhaps I paused from the reflective effort because the leadership module on quality was less reflective in its nature. It wasn't until the last two taught modules on chaos theory and alternative perspectives on leadership that I stepped upon my steepest learning curve. Even though I had thought I was reflecting on a deep level, I wasn't. My reflections had tended to be looking out rather than looking in. My progress to becoming mindful in practice had been minimal. Looking back, I could see that my reflections had been superficial. I really began to see myself as the leader I was – essentially transactional. I also began to see that if I wanted to be transformational it had to start with me. This sounds obvious but I had been conforming to type, somehow believing that theory alone would rationally change me. My guide's exhortations had fallen on deaf ears! Senge's words (1990: 173) were a wake-up call: 'Actions always speak louder than words. There is nothing more powerful I can do to influence others than to seriously pursue my own desire to be a personal mater.'

Following this came the dramatic revelation that this was a lifelong journey. There was no Oz! I had to focus on the journey, not the outcome. I had to discover the art of holding creative tension in my practice. The next wake-up call was academically failing two modules. It was as if I had been caught in no-man's-land between a transactional and a transformational approach to writing. I was trying to write transformationally without being transformational, entangled again in the literature. What I wrote just didn't make sense. It reflected my confusion. It may have been easier to throw in the towel but I do persist in hard times – one transformational characteristic I was well endowed with. I had to let go of my effort to control the learning process. My reflections led me to challenge more deeply my mental models that lay beneath the surface of my behaviour. I realised this was the key to learning. Yet unearthing them was no easy task.

Likes status quo (likes to be in control)	Constraining mental models (seeing reality for what it is)	
Fuzzy vision		
Conflict avoider (no possibility of learning)	Poor reflective skills (no insight into self)	Literature in my head not in my heart

Stemming from unearthing my mental models, reinforced my insight that I liked order, stability and predictability was reinforced. Undertaking the chaos theory module brought me head to head with these traits, grounded as they were in Newtonian thinking. I had to admit that chaos, despite its affinity with transformational leadership, was my antithesis. The word 'chaos' conjures up what, in my Newtonian world, I fear most: disruption, confusion and loss of control. Rationally I could not accept that order is patterned within chaos.

The contradiction was stark, forcing me to confront what type of leader I really wanted to be. I thought I was emancipated but I was still shackled to transactional thinking. I learnt some hard truths. I wrote in my diary:

I thought today, how would I cope without the degree of control I am used to, allowing chaos into my life ... scary, very scary! I realise I hate it when I am not in control. And yet I see that chaos is true. It makes sense.

I faced Schuster's two leadership attributes[4] that most defined me as transactional:

- You can share power with others. You believe that sharing power is the best way to tap talent, engage others and finish the task in optimal fashion.
- Your character is well developed without the prominent dark side of ego power. People trust that you are as you seem because your behaviour aligns with your words.

Through my reflections I came to see myself as chaos inside, not outside. I learnt that I sought control out there because I was not in control inside me. Such insight was revelatory. I could see the way I projected my insecurity onto others, into the environment. I came to see that the need to control reflects weak power whereas letting go of the need to control was truly powerful. All my professional life I had unwittingly been conforming, allowing myself to be controlled. Chaos is liberating. I am a whole person. I evince a concern for my wholeness. Can I see ME through the mist of delusions?

I felt exactly as Wheatley (1999: 168) writes: 'Like all journeys, this one moves through both the dark and light, the terrors of the unknown and the joys of deep recognition. Some shapes and landmarks are already clear. Others wait to be discovered. No one can say where the journey is leading. But the relationship promises to be fruitful, and I can feel the explorer's blood rising in me. I am glad to feel in awe again.'

Likes status quo (likes to conform and be in control)	Constraining mental models (seeing reality for it is is)	Realising the chaos inside me (my point of crisis and transition)
Fuzzy vision	ME	Accepting the nature of my current reality as unsatisfactory
Conflict avoider (no possibility of learning)	Poor reflective skills (no insight into self)	Literature in my head not in my heart

So the final parts of my puzzle were positioned. My journey so far, rather disappointingly, and quite opposite to my optimistic forecast, had found me to be largely transactional. Yet I had truly internalised that I wanted to be a transformational leader. The challenge, in the time left, was to make this a reality. I felt I had moved into a clearing of self-knowing, understanding my current reality where I could truly hold creative tension. I had no need to be defensive anymore, supported by peers and guides within the guided reflection group.

I even wrote a poem:

> Busy doing, beavering away
> I've forgotten my purpose in my busy days.
> What's important, what makes me stay?
> Why do I come here day after day?
>
> To ensure that the patients get only the best
> that care is best quality that they'll ever get.
> My purpose is to ensure this is always true
> through developing and guiding and welcoming the new.
>
> My vision is of a harmonious team
> working together, motivated and keen
> of patients and relatives who all have a voice,
> of patients allowed to make their own choice.
>
> Of evidence-based care given as course,
> of dignity and humanity practised at source,
> of a unit whose reputation spreads far and wide
> for its quality of care for others as a guide.
>
> Where staff know what's right and how to act,
> where the best for patients is their only pact,
> the patient and family always at the heart
> this is the place from which it all starts.

I had journeyed along the leadership path for 18 months to reach this point. Of course my journey was not quite as linear as I present it in the puzzle. The puzzle does offer a vivid picture of my transactional embodiment and how that picture constrained me from realising my desired way of being. I learnt that such embodiment is reinforced daily by normal patterns of relating grounded in power and tradition. Now, after 18 months, I had a more authentic grasp of my current reality as the basis for stepping further along the road. Now I shifted to reflect on a series of experiences that affirmed my movement towards realising transformational leadership reflected in a new set of congruent mental models.

A guided reflection session found me saying that I didn't have anything to reflect on. I said that everything was fine at work. Inevitably I was challenged.

It was again suggested I still liked the status quo, keeping it easy, conforming rather than challenging. I went home despondent.

Ruffled, I wrote in my journal: 'What's wrong with that?'

At the next group session I was again challenged. Was I in a comfort zone, following normative patterns, is everything fine, are we all happy, don't we rock the boat? I almost screamed, *YES. What's wrong with that?*

Instinctively I said nothing; it's easy, it's fine, I'm happy … but am I? NO! I need to start living what I have learnt in my head and make it real. So the plan tomorrow is that I am going to try and be mindful in all that I do and spend time reflecting on what I do … watch this space!

I wrote another poem, turning my despondency into energy:

My difficulty in being mindful

My difficulty in being mindful is that my mind is always full!
Kids and work, house and life all exert their pull,
dawn to dusk don't stop to think, don't let the demons in,
just keep on going, get tasks done, too busy to hear the din
to pause a while and clear my head is a scary place to be
being quiet and relax are never really me
I get uncomfortable, feel disturbed, if I get too deep
perhaps I fear being mindful will only lose me sleep.

I used to be a thoughtful soul, always questioned why,
wrote my thoughts in rhyme or prose allowed my soul to fly
I was violated, read, exposed, vowed never again no more
emotions ceased, thoughts dried up, experience too raw
my fear is not of losing sleep but opening up my soul
but now it's time to try again, the journey being my goal
I fear emotion, I fear myself, I fear that I will change
and yet this is the ultimate aim, I want to try again.
I dare myself to explore, myself, my thoughts, my heart
to make being mindful a skilled part off my craft
here's to trying …

I realised I had a minefield of material to reflect on. The earlier gradual realisation that it had to begin with ME started to truly hit home.

ME

I'd reached a point where I was absorbing the literature, making it real for me. I actually found myself thinking today, how would someone who practises Schuster's philosophy have reacted? Slowly but surely I was reflecting more naturally and becoming more mindful of self as a leader. Today, I deliberately made myself stop and think and it did help me see things more clearly. If I had just ploughed on in my normal way, I think I would have been unprofessional, rude and probably made the wrong decision.

ME	
Being mindful of self within practice	Holding a vision of leadership

At this time, I undertook the Myers–Briggs Type Indicator test, emerging as an introvert (I), intuitive (N), thinker (T) judger (J). INTJs are inclined to focus on their own inner thoughts and abstract ideas and often prefer working on their own. Quietly curious and introspective, they are inclined to focus on the deeper patterns and hidden meanings behind the surface forms and structures. They tend to view life from a somewhat detached, academic point of view. Logical, analytical and orderly in their thinking, they are motivated to get to the heart of theoretical issues. Having a strong sense of responsibility, they believe it is important to adhere closely to established methods and procedures. However, their emphasis on thinking may cause them to question tasks and procedures that are not based on sound logical analysis. As Smathers (2005) noted, rather than engaging in lively, informed debate or discussion, they will generally prefer to learn about a subject by reading or through private study. I recognise that these are the mental models that thwart me – perhaps an answer to the question as to why I found reflection so challenging. As an introvert, I am not inclined to share easily. As a thinker I prefer logical analysis to feelings, and although I can reflect continually in the privacy of my own mind, I find it difficult to expose these thoughts to others. I prefer to judge situations rather than perceive their meaning and, due to my introverted nature, I am not inclined to write down my thoughts. These traits combined to make me reluctant to confront conflict, preferring to be in control and be controlled, in my safe haven, conforming to what is expected. My introvert nature allows me to be oppressed and in turn, an oppressor. It's been a struggle, a conscious effort, scary, exposing and frightening, but I know I can move forward. The transformation begins.

I was keeping hold of my vision when confronted with reality, holding creative tension. It was as if someone had opened a door for me to see myself moment by moment. It was liberating and remarkably powerful. It gave me a new sense of control that I have never known before. My guide had said, 'transformational leadership was powerful'. Now I could feel it. The next issue was to dust off my vision and make it shine again, and infuse my colleagues with it. We began to move from a task-oriented practice to a more values-oriented practice where we began to dialogue about our practice, being more critical and open to new ideas. In doing so we built a new sense of community within our practice. Moving from ME to WE.

Vibrant, alive, vision Building community – a shift to WE	ME	
A shared and vibrant vision	Being mindful of self within practice	Holding a real vision of leadership

So I finally took the risk and made an important decision. I learnt that risk taking can and does work and could be rather enjoyable. I am learning that other staff, when given the chance, can take on responsibility and do it well. It became my lot to help Louisa, a sister on the unit who was not performing well enough. I groaned inwardly at the thought. Yet I was positive and helped her see herself as others saw her and take responsibility. I could see how my mental models affected me, and to my surprise my mental models shifted and I was able to feel compassion and empathy. I learnt my mental models could be overcome once acknowledged. Working with Louisa, I could see her difficulties were also linked to her mental models and vision. Refocusing these in tune with her own leadership as a unit sister became the focus for our learning together.

Transforming mental models	Risks, experiments and learns	
Vibrant, alive, vision Building a community – a shift to WE	ME	
Holding creative tension	Being mindful of self within practice	Holding a real vision of leadership

I wrote in my dairy:

> Today I realised that I have stopped making lists and sometimes I even forget to look in my diary, as doing everything is no longer so important to me. I constantly get interrupted and it all changes so quickly but actually I don't mind. I am definitely learning to let go. I think this has been helped by being acting matron as well as my normal role in that I am now having to let go of some things in order to stay afloat. However, the knock-on effect of that is I am learning to share power with others

and that, given the opportunity, staff can and do rise to the occasion. Situations just seem to work out better that way.

I would never have described myself as a control freak and yet looking back I can sense how I needed to control situations as a way of controlling my inherent anxiety, as if I don't quite trust more junior staff to make good decisions. I know the buck stops with me! As such, letting go of the need to control everything was not easy. It's also risky if staff are not developed or supported enough. As a leader I must be a role model and teacher, an investor in people and relationships.

My engagement with chaos theory marked a huge shift in my perspective on leadership. It taught me that practice is inherently chaotic (hence my anxiety!) and yet chaos is a positive force because things are essentially unpredictable and uncertain in health care situations. It is about trusting my instincts and intuitive sense of what's going on. In the language of chaos theory, my leadership and practice visions are strange attractors around which order is governed as we move through the situation. The right things just happen! From a chaos perspective I could also appreciate the idea of foresight – seeing situations before they occurred rather than reacting to them. A new paradoxical order manifests itself that is far more satisfying for all staff in contrast with the command and control style that had typified my previous management. This shift was not easy and yet one day it happened I could feel the tension release itself from me. Wheatley (1999: 119) writes, 'it is chaos' great destructive energy that dissolves the past and gives us the gift of a new future. It releases us from the imprisoning patterns of the past by offering us its wild ride into newness. Only chaos creates the abyss in which we can create ourselves.' Hang on tight!

Risks, experiments and learns	Mindful of mental models	Embracing chaos (letting go of control)
Vibrant, alive, vision Building a community – a shift to WE	ME	
Holding creative tension	Being mindful of self within practice	Holding a real vision of leadership

Just one square of the puzzle remained. A situation occurred on the unit that involved conflict with one of the consultants over changing an aspect of practice he was vehemently against. I was able to challenge him and challenge my own conformist self, revealing the real reasons for his resistance and securing his agreement. Most importantly, I realised I could challenge the consultant. I didn't have to conform to what others wanted. I had used the creative tension and taken on the most difficult man and got the guideline agreed. And yes, it felt good and yet it wasn't an ego thing. I was thinking and feeling collaborative. I think he sensed this because normally he would have competed until he won. He views me differently now, with more respect even if at times grudgingly. Leopards do not so much lose their spots but they can be repatterned.

Risks, experiments and learns	Mindful of mental models	Chaos versus control
Vibrant, alive, vision Building a community – a shift to WE	ME	Collaborator (no longer the conformist caught up on ego)
Holding creative tension	Being mindful of self within practice	Holding a real vision of leadership

I feel I am still at the beginning of something. My jigsaw now looks more the way I want it to look, but all these attributes are in their infancy and need honing, maturing. My challenge is to keep moving forward on my lifelong discovery of transformational leadership. I find myself not wanting to write a conclusion or summary of my insights. I don't feel there is one. I have learnt this journey is never ending. I know that the journey of being and becoming is not predictable and that there is no solution to be found out there for becoming a transformational leader. Transformational leadership is about the person I am, not the techniques I might learn.

That sounds so obvious now, yet, as I have written, for much of the time I just didn't get it. I still have to learn more about going to the edge, gaining confidence that creativity lies there, and away from the apparent safety of conformity. I am getting closer. I am also confident that I do not have to fear falling over the edge. Transformational leadership by its very nature is chaotic; it is like life itself, eminently unpredictable. Yet being mindful, holding a true vision, having confidence in my ability, being true to myself, I have nothing to fear. Indeed, the very uncertainty of practice is its creative turn that I embrace with enthusiasm. I have talked with other group members about meeting regularly to reflect and support each other. I sense this is vital. I sense how easily it might be to slip back into previously learnt ways when the new ways are vulnerable and not strongly embedded.

Reflecting on the modern matron role. It certainly sharpened my sense of leadership from the perspective of managing the unit although, in hindsight, I could see more clearly the way my CPD (continuing professional development) role was positionally grounded in my expert and persuasive power qualities (French and Raven 1968) as I had no line management relationships except from the old modern matron!

Ideas come and go. Some ideas come around again in the search for meaning and utility. One such idea is the matron. Modern matrons were introduced by the NHS plan in order to provide unambiguous, visible leadership on the wards in response to public demand. The Department of Health document *Nearly 2000 modern matrons in the NHS – Two years early* (2001b: 2) states, 'Matrons will be accountable for a group of wards; they will be easily identifiable to patients, highly visible, accessible and authoritative figures to whom patients and their families can turn for assistance, advice and support and upon whom they can rely on to ensure that the fundamentals of care are right backed up by appropriate administrative support'.

To ensure that the fundamentals of care are right reads like the remit of a quality policewoman. Troubleshooting to nip trouble in the bud. No mention of leadership in these words. The Department of Health document (2003) *Modern matrons – Improving the patient experience* lists the modern matron's ten key responsibilities:

- Leading by example
- Making sure patients get quality care
- Ensuring staffing is appropriate to patient needs
- Empowering staff to take on a wide range of clinical tasks
- Improving hospital cleanliness
- Ensuring patients' nutritional needs are met
- Improving wards for patients
- Making sure patients are treated with respect
- Preventing hospital-acquired infection
- Resolving problems for patients and their relatives by building closer relationships

Whilst this list of duties has a strong sense of ensuring quality, it has at least some words associated with leadership – leading by example and empowering staff. When I have discussed these responsibilities with modern matrons they shrug their shoulders. They say it is like trying to patch a huge crack with filler and hope that nobody notices that the building is actually collapsing. Empowering staff to do more when the staff are already stretched may feel more akin to bullying than empowering.

The word 'matron' itself is deeply symbolic of an authoritative tradition that demanded subordination. It is symbolic of the chasm between organisational reality and leadership ideal. Fundamentally, matron leadership has to be concerned with creating a healthy work environment that benefits patients and staff – a workplace that is humanised in contrast with the dehumanising toxic environment of the transactional organisation that sees everyone as objects to be manipulated towards achieving outcomes. Yet accommodated into the transactional organisational machine, the matron role becomes primarily concerned with smoothing out organisational anxiety. Early evaluation reports (commissioned by the Department of Health (2004a)) indicate a huge variation in these roles across the country. They warn that in the absence of adequate time or resources there is a danger of 'the potential of these posts being squandered' (Duffin and Lipley 2005: 7). Generally, evaluation of the modern matron role is uncertain from published studies (Ashman et al. 2006.). In one audit of the role (Dealey et al. 2007), measured against agreed corporate objectives and utilising questionnaires sent to all senior nurses and a range of trust staff, the researchers note, 'Senior nurses were found to be satisfied with their role and the preparation for and understanding of their role seemed to be successful. There were many improvements such as a reduction in drug errors, complaints and MRSA bacteriaemias.' They conclude that the implementation of the *modern matron* role has been successful and made improvements in patient care. The many improvements seem related to smooth running rather than leadership. I can't say the modern matron role is successful. It is added pressure to ensure outcomes, especially related to infection control, creating an illusion that something is being done about it to reassure the public.

Conclusion

The idea of Lisa deconstructing herself and then reconstructing herself is more dynamic than the jigsaws suggests. The developmental time of 18 months to reach the moment of transition is significant. It indicates, as with all the leadership narratives, that it takes time and dedicated support to become a true leader especially when working in transactional organisations where the aspiring leader can feel isolated. Given the organisational environment, such leadership is precarious, suggesting that organisations, if they are to take leadership seriously, need to actively support aspiring leaders within practice. Such journeys cannot be rushed although the pressure to realise leadership can become stressful and counterproductive.

Lisa's revelation of 'poor reflective skills' is a common factor for leaders engaging in reflection in any depth. Most leaders had experienced reflective teaching but this had tended to be superficial, scratching at the surface of experience. It had no depth. Perhaps one reason for avoiding depth is the ontological sense of becoming. It is self-revealing. It may be uncomfortable but it is vital.

Reflection

Perhaps now is the time to start your own leadership journey.

Step 1 – Try writing a leadership vision however tentative.

Step 2 – Write a description of an experience that says something about living this leadership vision. To help you, use the model for structured reflection (Figure A1.1 – Appendix 1). Try and explore the depth of the cues. Be patient. It is your life. It is your journey.

Step 3 – What insights do you gain? How do these insights impact on your future practice? You will know this by reflecting on similar experiences.

Step 4 – Find someone within your organisation who is also interested in becoming a leader. Create a community and guide each other through your experiences.

Notes

1. From 2000 to 2006 Nigel Crisp was Permanent Secretary of the UK Department of Health and Chief Executive of the English NHS – the biggest health organisation in the world with 1.3 million employees – where he led major reforms. He described these in *24 Hours to Save the NHS – the Chief Executive's Account of Reform 2000 to 2006* and draws out the lessons for the future. He argues that further radical reform is needed if the NHS is to remain affordable and sustainable and that other countries can learn from the experience in England. I couldn't trace the context of his quoted words. www.nigelcrisp.com.
2. By collaborative, Lisa refers to Thomas and Kilmann's conflict mode instrument (see Figure 4.2).
3. See Figure 2.1.
4. See Figure 2.1.

8 The Bubble in the Machine

The good traveller

As I have shown through the narratives, becoming a leader is a unique journey and yet there are many similarities because of the shared visions of leadership and the transactional culture of health care organisations. Because of this shared background it has been possible to understand something of the nature of becoming a mindful leader within health care organisations or, for that matter, within any organisation.

The mindful leader is a good traveller. 'A good traveller has no fixed plans and is not intent on arriving' (Tzu 1999).[1] She chooses her own path even though well-worn paths may offer an easier ascent and may be helped as necessary by guides, mindful of every step, paying attention and appreciating the journey (Pirsig 1974). She sets her own pace, yet mindful of not being left behind. She ensures her support knowing that the path might be rough, littered with pitfalls and hazards. Lather (1993: 674) describes that practice can be 'a broken and uneven place, heavily inscribed with habit and sedimented relationships'.

The good traveller puts down her old transactional baggage and lightens up, freeing herself to wear her new leadership clothes. She engages patiently in constant dialogue with other travellers and with appropriate guidebooks to inform the journey. She is intuitive, traversing the indeterminate complex lowlands of professional practice (Schön 1987).

There are no prescribed solutions or formulas that can be applied to solve the problems that face leaders in everyday situations. All situations require careful understanding and judgement as to how to respond the best. Pinar (1981: 180–1) reinforces the significance of intuition: 'All knowing begins in intuition. It is the medium through which the qualities of situation become discerned, conceptualised and articulated. Intuition is the representation and mediation of the situation and self. Thus, it behoves us to be interested in knowing how to cultivate the intuitive capacity, and to begin to utilise language to render our intuitions sensitively, hence more accurately.'

The good traveller is both artist and scientist; the good artist uses empathy whereas the good scientist uses reason. Both are valuable ways of knowing (Belenky et al. 1986).[2] The leader synchronises these ways of knowing and finds the right balance. Becoming mindful, the leader begins to see situations for what they are with poise, able to weigh up each situation on its merits, and respond with foresight always mindful of creating and sustaining community. The good traveller is a bubble in the machine.

The bubble in the machine

Through guiding leaders over the past 12 years I know that the transactional pyramid is not easily shifted. As such, the leader becomes the bubble in the machine, a metaphoric virus infecting the transactional organisation with his or her leadership values, protected by a wall of mindfulness.

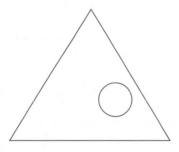

When leaders are connected within organisations the virus spreads more quickly, moving towards critical mass when the shape of the pyramid itself begins to transform. The bubble expands to fill the organisational space, transforming people as it touches them. The bubble is irresistible because it is good and compelling. The bubble is community, a playground, a laboratory, a dialogical space, a greenhouse, an energy converter and a generator. It is an inspirer where the leader holds creative tension and where every step is purposeful to realising leadership and as a consequence a flourishing of the organisation. Gradually, leadership repatterns organisational relationships around shared values and shared success. It rips up the transactional motif of smooth running.

Leadership actively seeks to disturb smooth running in its quest to establish more effective practice by treading the creative edge between equilibrium and disequilibrium. Mycek (1999: 13) writes '"We are living on an edge", says Leland Kaiser.' 'It is an edge between two eras, two cultural mind-sets, two ways of doing things. Edges have fascinating possibilities. Some people approach the edge, become fearful and retreat to the safety of an old and familiar surface. Other people get reckless and fall off the edge into despair and ruin. A few brave travellers use the edge as a platform to leap into new possibilities. These few travellers are the way-makers for the next century. They lay down the pathway for others to follow.' 'On the edge, you take responsibility for the creation of your preferred reality,' he continues. 'You understand that universe will support you 100% and you embrace chaos as unlimited opportunity. Your imagination becomes your tool of creation. You are as limited as it is, but no more so.'

Myceck's paper entitled 'Teetering on the Edge of Chaos' is a fitting metaphor for the journey of being and becoming a leader within the prevailing transactional health care organisations. Leadership is embracing and dancing with chaos, in the sense that the leader knows that nothing is certain, yet knowing that order manifests itself around meaning. The shift from being transactional to being transformational is chaotic. It is not a known logical linear path of acquiring skills. It is an ontological process of becoming that involves unlearning transactional ways of seeing and responding that are deeply embodied and reinforced in daily patterns of relating. The leadership path lies within each leader. It is a path that requires vision, imagination and creativity. However, leaders can stumble and fall. At times, especially at the beginning of the journey, the emerging leaders are anxious and hang onto embodied transactional ways of being as if they were mooring posts. Feeling vulnerable and insecure they seek comfort in the familiar where nothing changes except their frustration. Then the support of a leadership community is vital.

Working through creative tension

The transactional pyramid resists a transformational/servant leadership type of leadership because it is culture shock. Indeed, you are probably wondering whether mindful leadership *can* be realised within the transactional culture of health care organisations given the inevitable resistance to it. This vexing question must be of prime concern to anyone who recognises that real leadership is the greatest concern and hope for better health care organisations.

Leaders surf the creative tension, weathering the stormy waves that threaten to submerge them. In doing so they learn to weigh up and yield diplomatically to resistance. Better to yield than drown. Yielding is not failure; it is a vital attribute of leadership. Yielding is a political game, recognising that asserting leadership is a fine line to tread along the corridors of power. The astute game player does not marginalise self. Leaders chip away at the dominant transactional culture. They throw their hands in the air with frustration and seemingly smack their heads against hard walls. But they do make an impact within themselves and within the teams in which they work. Rather like climbing uphill with a rucksack full of stones. Slowly the stones are discarded one by one and the climb becomes easier. Just reflect, learn, smile and get back on the surfboard.

It becomes a question of integrity. Remen (2000: 53) captures the significance of integrity: 'Sometimes we live in ways that are too small, and in places that focus and develop only a part of who we are. When we do, the life in us may become squeezed into a shape that is not our own. We may not even realise that this is so. Despite this, something deep in us that holds our integrity inviolate will find ways to remind us of the breath and depth of life in us and assert its wholeness.'

Become squeezed into a shape that is not our own reflects Alison's sense of being put in her place.[3] To reiterate, transformational/servant leadership and transactional leadership are essentially different ways of being in the world. Holding creative tension, aspiring leaders learn to appreciate the culture of the transactional organisation and how it constrains realising desired leadership. As leaders became more mindful of themselves as leaders, they more easily recognise creative tension when their behaviour does not align with their words. It is always a potent challenge – 'Do I walk the talk?'

Shifting norms

The shift to creating a culture of leadership can be viewed as a series of contrasting social norms (Table 8.1) that helps the leader to visualise creative tension. I have grouped transformational and servant leadership together although there are obviously differences between them with which the reader will have become cognisant. The norms are linked within a whole. As such, a shift within one norm inevitably ripples through all of them. The ripple inevitably triggers a response to reassert smooth running. However, smooth running is an illusion simply because the organisation is in perpetual crisis reacting to its poor functioning. That in itself is perceived as normal and therefore not a problem. It is as if the transactional world is devoid of wisdom as it lurches from pillar to post.

In a rational world people would simply shift norms to become leaders. But life is not rational. Barriers to rational change are authority or force, tradition and embodiment (Fay 1987). Shifting norms is profoundly difficult simply because norms govern everyday practice and are embodied in

Transactional culture	Creative tension					Transformational/servant leader culture
	1	2	3	4	5	
Vision (often postulated as a mission statement) is set 'on high' and transmitted down the hierarchical pyramid written in corporate speak and rhetoric influenced by external agendas.						Vision is set collaboratively (around the table) by people who work together within the organisation and who are cognisant of external agendas.
Structured through a rigid set of hierarchical rungs that define role and authority. At each level, the pyramidal shape of the organisation is replicated. Management rules, okay!						Structured through a collaborative network of local units with a strong degree of self-determination (flattened hierarchy) and powerful leadership.
High level of anxiety to meet its organisational objectives transmitted down through the strata of hierarchy. This leads to a strong sense of compliance and conformity.						Low level of anxiety due to genuine patterns of collaborative relationships working together towards shared success. This leads to a strong sense of commitment and motivation.
Views problems as threats to the organisation's primary goal of its own smooth running. Care is secondary (blame-and-shame culture).						Views problems as positive learning opportunities (risks/experiments and learns).
Views people in terms of tasks to be done in exchange for reward – extrinsic motivators of reward. Staff do not feel valued.						Invests in people to unleash talent and intellectually stimulate – intrinsic motivators of reward. Staff feel valued.

Emphasis on force (command and control), especially authoritative power (thin trust/high fear/insecurity).	Emphasis on devolving power, especially facilitative power (thick trust/low fear/insecurity).
Relationships with subordinates characterised by parent–child patterns of relating (from a transactional analysis perspective) (views people as essentially irresponsible).	Relationships with colleagues characterised by adult–adult patterns of relating (from a transactional analysis perspective) (views people as essentially responsible).
Single feedback loops to monitor objectives being met and maintain the status quo. This approach views the organisation as essentially mechanical where parts are viewed in isolation of the whole. Change tends to be reactive to fix emerging problems (Newtonian/reductionist perspective).	Double feedback loops to monitor both process and outcome and the relationship between them. This approach views the organisation as a whole and the relationships within it as dynamic and evolving (chaos theory/holistic perspective).
Emphasis on management (either passive or active) that is reactive, oppressive and mindless.	Emphasis on leadership that is proactive, enabling, moral and mindful.
Staff are socialised to 'know your place' within the organisation to ensure its smooth running (self-regulation based on fear).	Staff are enabled to 'be in-place, for optimum performance and self-realisation (self-liberation based on aspiration).

Table 8.1 The movement from transactional to transformational social norms

everyday relationships. People have learnt to be transactional and that the transactional world isn't going to shift easily. As Wedderburn-Tate (1999) suggests, for someone with a predominantly transactional style of leadership, adopting transformative skills is extremely difficult.

To unlearn self in an environment that constantly demands conformity to learnt ways is undoubtedly difficult. The leader takes on a dual personality, undermining the old and empowering the new, like trying to strip off a tightly fitting suit whilst simultaneously trying on a new suit. Norms, if understood correctly, can be chipped away like a sculptor crafting a fine piece of art. As the leader chips away, the vision becomes more formed. Others can see and feel its momentum. As such, shifts gather momentum.

Table 8.1 might be written in many different ways. I am certain there are norms that I have not identified or could be written differently. Consider the veracity of these norms within your practice. Mark on the 1–5 scale to construct a graph where you think your organisation is. As a leader, where would you start to shift norms? Perhaps start by becoming mindful of transactional analysis and consciously move into adult–adult relationships with others.[4] How do others respond? How do you feel? Use the mantra 'Tough on the issues, soft on the people' to see problems as learning opportunities to counter the oppressive blame-and-shame culture that characterises high-anxiety organisations.

The transactional paradigm does seem to reflect the all-pervasive frame of reference that is fundamental to the received wisdom on strategic management in the NHS. A brief glance at the current strategic vision for the NHS would seem to betray an adherence to the belief that target setting, performance monitoring, time framing and firm top-down management are the desirable mechanistic and scientific methodologies for advancement of the service evidenced by a raft of official plans, frameworks and policies. Elements of health service management and leadership such as carefully planned and enforced three-year nursing strategies, monitored adherence to job descriptions, performance appraisal, core expected behaviours and clinical supervision conducted from a technical rather than emancipatory stance, all point to a pervasive heavily transactional culture in the NHS (Johns 2003). Conversely, harking back to the *Making a difference* document, it exhorts nurses to become leaders who establish direction and purpose, inspire, motivate and empower teams around common goals – leaders who are motivated, self-aware, socially skilled and collaborative (Department of Health 1999). These qualities seem more apposite to the transformational leadership approach and the potential for tension between such nurse leaders and the prevailing transactional culture of the NHS appears all too evident. The professed desire of the government to create a professional and organisational climate that enables nurse leaders to challenge orthodoxy, take risks and learn from experience seems in danger of being accused of empty rhetoric.

Perhaps there is a middle way, whereby the best qualities of the transactional and transformational/servant leadership are synergised. Marquis and Huston (1996) comment that although the transformational leader is held as the current ideal, the transactional qualities of the day-to-day managerial role are still important. This perspective suggests that both transformational and transactional qualities need to be present in the same individual in varying degrees. They argue that the leader needs to tread with extreme caution to ensure that the critical balance is maintained. The problem with this position is that the transactional will always be dominant because of existing norms. A different view is that the transactional is subsumed within the transformational, simply because the leader is always a skilled manager and always works towards synergy.

Becoming a leader is a shift from an essentially product-governed world to a process world. This is not to say products, targets, outcomes, call them whatever – they fundamentally stem from the same mindset, no matter how management attempts to package them – are not necessary to some extent. It is the emphasis that shifts. Wheatley (1999: 154) reflects the significance of this shift: 'But the greatest challenge for me lies not in adopting any one new method, but in learning generally to live in a process world. It's a completely new way to be. Life demands that I participate with things as they unfold, to expect to be surprised, to honour the mystery of it, and see what emerges. These were difficult lessons to learn. I was well-trained to create things – plans, events, measures, programs. I invested more than half my life in trying to make the world conform to what I thought was best for it. It's not easy to give up the role of master creator and move into the dance of life.'

Mary writes: The leadership programme has transformed me from being a transactional manager into a transformational leader. Although as a manager I believed I led with a transformational flavour, you had to get deep down and peep through the keyhole to see it. I have learnt along my journey that leadership is much more than being taught; it is learning, and that the leader keeps learning (Vail 1996) and continuously facilitates learning around those with whom she works. Learning has become natural for me as I have become more mindful of myself as a leader. It is a simple equation.

(Continued)

My journey from a transactional manager to transformational leader has been a journey from darkness into light. It has not been easy. I have struggled with many difficult feelings and extreme emotions that I have never experienced before. I had an ongoing internal battle that raged as I grappled at leadership theories and the reality of how I was going to manage the service – weaving management within my leadership in congruent ways. 'The Service' was my baby! I had nurtured it from infancy into this huge and increasingly complex organisation. But as I grew along the journey and embraced the wider culture of the PCT, being told to conform to the PCT's transactional culture, the frustration I felt was immense. I have struggled with the tension of my current reality and my vision of where and who I would like to be. Now, looking back I can see my reflexive journey with astonishing clarity. I truly feel liberated and transformed and recognise that the service too has been transformed for the better. I honestly feel that if I had not completed this course, I would no longer be manager of 'The Service'. Before embarking on the programme, the joy had gone out of my life and I was just going through the motions. This would eventually have been too much and I would have abandoned my vision in favour of sanity. There is always a transactional price to pay of not conforming! That would have been such a waste and would have left me leaving a failure and regretful. Wheatley (1999) suggests that if I believe that, as a leader, I must have my hands into everything, controlling every decision, every person and every moment, then I cannot hope for anything except what I already have – a treadmill of frantic effort that would ultimately result in destroying myself and the collective vitality with those who I work with. It was certainly going that way. The bigger 'The Service' became the more frantic I became. It was so insidious I didn't see it creeping up. 'The Service' has blossomed into a thriving, innovative service. I have been able to let go of my stranglehold and empower others to take responsibility and thrive. I know I will always surface challenges to the way I lead as others' actions make me anxious from time to time. Yet being mindful I can see myself more clearly. Smile instead of frown and see the anxious moment as a learning moment. Yet such lessons have been difficult to learn wrapped up in the moment. Coming to the community of inquiry, I can tell the story and see it, and slowly I began to resolve the tension within practice. I have opened my existing windows wider and opened windows I didn't know existed to see an amazing landscape full of possibilities. I now live leadership. It is transparent.

(Continued)

Glouberman (2003) suggests we live in a culture where we are valued more for what we achieve in the eyes of others than what we achieve in our own eyes. I feel good when people acknowledge what has been achieved. It has not been easy to let go of control and have others received acclaim for their work. But giving power away has given me the freedom to explore other possibilities that I could only have ever dreamed about and I would never have had the courage to take these dreams forward. In letting go of control I have learnt that things evolve and pattern around vision and intent. I now see a future full of exciting possibilities! I relate very much to Glouberman's idea of spending much of my previous life as a manager as a rat on an exercise wheel in a cage, trying to keep up with the inner and outer expectations that dominated my life. Every now and then I kicked the exercise wheel or rattled the bars of the cage but doing this just delayed me; eventually I would go back to the wheel, running faster to make up for lost time. Whatever I did, whether it was something I really wanted to do or something I didn't, the inner result was just the same: even my most creative desires were transformed into expectations that ended up oppressing me. I was constantly trying to do too much! This is not the end of my journey; my journey is now a lifelong commitment that I undertake in my quest to be a true leader. It has given new meaning to my life, my role as manager and the service as a whole. Such was the vitality of the community of learning that we plan to continue to meet. We have formed a strong bond that can never be broken.

Where now?

Efforts to develop leadership have largely been instrumental, grounded in the dominant values of the transactional culture that characterises NHS health care organisations despite the call for a more enlightened view of leadership. The rhetoric around leadership is evidenced within contemporary leadership literature and Department of Health white papers. However such rhetoric falls flat for two key reasons. Firstly, the NHS culture cannot accommodate genuine leadership. Accommodation theory suggests that ideal models will always be distorted to fit the prevailing culture (Latimer 1995). Secondly, the idea of leadership is poorly understood because it is viewed from a transactional perspective.

I must be optimistic that mindful leadership programmes can transform the transactional organisation to liberate staff at every level of the organisation to deliver effective and humanised care. The narratives suggest the possibility.

Janet writes: I worry that I may lose momentum after the leadership programme is over, perhaps even lose direction, yet I am comforted by the knowledge that I now easily hold creative tension. It is part of who I now am. My world has shifted, my perspectives altered and my consciousness raised. I am more aware and analytical of the ways in which the past influences me now in my thoughts and feelings.

I am more often either the lone voice at meetings supporting change, or the one who is truly listening, suspending judgement, without any personal agenda beyond seeking the most effective practice. I am mindful of being 'of service' to others even when they resist or rebut me. I am released to be able to practise in new ways and to influence others as I do so.

Community

Janet recognised the value of an ongoing supportive community. It should be relatively easy for her to create such a group within her organisation. After all, it is a quality of leadership. The benefits of this would enable both herself and others to reflect on and develop their leadership. Her organisation, having supported her to attend the programme, could establish ongoing support on a more formal basis, investing in the investment and enabling Janet's learning to ripple through the organisation. However, there was no evidence of such leadership initiatives. Why was that? It seems there is an organisational inertia with regard to leadership. This is not surprising given the lack of a leadership culture endemic within NHS organisations.

In a study (Johns 2003) I undertook with fifteen ward managers in an acute NHS hospital setting, I used individual guided reflection to develop their leadership.[5] Although this approach opened a learning space to develop self as a leader, with hindsight I considered a group approach would have been more beneficial to enable the ward managers to share their collective experience and create a network for ongoing support for each other and possibly become an empowered, collective force. It was a significant insight to realise how isolated leaders were within the organisation and how their development may have benefited more from group-guided reflection with their peers rather than individually guided reflection. The ward managers emerged as a subordinate and powerless workforce within the order of things. The reflective effort threw them against brick walls of unrealistic expectation where they inevitably failed. Individual supervision increased their anxiety, adding as it did another level of pressure, one that was fundamentally difficult to realise within the transactional organisational culture.

Leadership – desire or threat?

Without doubt, becoming a leader is vital work. Once the aspiring leaders sensed its significance, there could be no compromise. Becoming a leader becomes a moral crusade simply because leaders realise that the organisation's failure to fulfil their mandate to care is an unacceptable contradiction. Caring *is* the core business of health care based around the patient's experience. It is not enough to be mediocre because mediocrity causes suffering to staff and patients and costs money. Lack of leadership costs the organisation millions when its workforce is not valued or invested in. It is not difficult to see the poverty of practitioners' lives within the transactional organisation and its consequences on service delivery.

Reviewing the collective narratives I was struck by how the transactional culture is characterised by a lack of honesty and empathy, and that transactional relationships are characterised by wearing masks that hide real agendas. Letting the masks go is difficult and yet, as Rebecca illuminates, it is possible. Pia could understand the nature of her relationships with her managers but could not easily shift them, because her response within these relationships had become embodied. Therein lay the crux of her leadership – how could she move beyond these oppressive relationships that took her life blood? For leaders to resist the transactional culture was subversive and courageous because of its emphasis on positional and coercive force. Resistance led to understanding the nature of one's current reality. Of course this needed to be a true understanding if it was to be the basis for transforming self and realising vision of self as a leader. Hence the role of the community of inquiry to enable the person to see herself truly as far as this was possible. Yet for some leaders the organisational environment was so barren for developing leadership that I wondered at their capacity to persevere or even to develop leadership in any meaningful way.

Aspiring leaders lacked confidence because they had been socialised into subordination. This was particularly true of nurses in contrast with other health care professionals such as occupational therapists and dieticians. Of course this must be expected. Egos are weak and precious, easily bruised, reflecting Schuster's reference to *the dark side of ego power*. As Sacks reminds us (1990: xiv), 'In the study of our most complex sufferings and disorder we are compelled to scrutinise the deepest, darkest, and most fearful parts of ourselves, the parts we all strive to deny or not to see. The thoughts which are most difficult to grasp or express are those which touch on this forbidden region and reawaken in us our strongest denials and our most profound intuitions.'

Time spans

It takes time, patience, commitment and guidance to become a leader. It is a slow walk up the mountain. To reiterate Wheatley (1999: 130), 'we slowly become who we want to be'. No shortcuts. Time span is vital. In general, it takes 18 months for the aspiring leader to prise her self free from transactional embodiment and perhaps another ten months for leadership to take firm root. Even then, the new leaders are fragile and must create their own support communities to sustain and further enable their leadership. Persistence and resilience are qualities of leadership that need constant nurturing. Such understanding makes a mockery of three-day leadership programmes. Such time spans will cause investment consternation. In a reactive world, organisations want quick returns.

Shifting the bubble upwards and downwards

None of the leaders were part of a mentoring leadership within their organisations. How much easier would the leadership path be if organisations genuinely embraced leadership in ways such that it is not reduced to a furtive subculture? This requires the organisation to embrace a vision of mindful leadership beyond any rhetoric. Imagine if chief executives embraced the leadership programme and publicly celebrated the leaders' success. The chief executive and the board members would be mindful leaders leading in tune with genuine leadership values. They would establish the learning organisation at the highest level and cascade it into every level of the organisation. Their corporate vision would state something like 'We are a learning organisation that invests in every member of staff through genuine leadership to succeed in collective and personal aspiration.' Then leaders would have powerful role models within practice. Then the transformational bubble could descend from the top, liberating and ultimately flattening the whole pyramid, coalescing with the bubbles from within.

Communities need to be no more than ten people to enable effective dialogue, multidisciplined at different hierarchical levels. The key is expert guidance to remind people about dialogue and counter any power plays. From a multidisciplinary perspective, this helps break down discipline silo walls.

Managers recoil when I point the finger and accuse them of failing to lead and liberate professionals to care. I remind them not to be resistant to the truth and to be open to the possibilities of a new way.

The King's Fund and Center for Creative Leadership report's (*Developing collective leadership for health care*) (West et al. 2014) primary message states: 'The most important determinant of the development and maintenance of an organisation's culture is current and future leadership. Every interaction by every leader at every level shapes the emerging culture of an organisation.' The difficulty with this statement, as I have evidenced, is creating the necessary culture shift to accommodate leadership in the first place. The report advocates a collective leadership that resonates with the notion of community. It sets out some key messages about its nature:

- Collective leadership means everyone taking responsibility for the success of the organisation as a whole – not just for their own jobs or work area. This contrasts with traditional approaches to leadership, which have focused on developing individual capability while neglecting the need for developing collective capability or embedding the development of leaders within the context of the organisation they are working in.
- Collective leadership cultures are characterised by all staff focusing on continual learning and, through this, on the improvement of patient care. It requires high levels of dialogue, debate and discussion to achieve shared understanding about quality problems and solutions.
- Leaders need to ensure that all staff adopt leadership roles in their work and take individual and collective responsibility for delivering safe, effective, high-quality and compassionate care for patients and service users. Achieving this requires careful planning, persistent commitment and constant focus on nurturing leadership and culture.

This rhetoric is compelling. Yet how to make it a reality? It is a clarion call for a mindful leadership guided over time. There is no quick fix. It is no good the CQC (Care Quality Commission) or Monitor adding 'leadership' to their quality tick list. That simply demands a reactive organisational response to comply on the surface whilst much of the underlying culture that resists such collective leadership remains essentially unchallenged, despite the recognition that it must not simply be challenged but changed.

Looking across the Atlantic towards the USA, I note that leadership in health care is facing some difficulty. Swensen et al. (2013) write, 'Leaders at all levels in care delivery organizations, not just senior executives, are struggling with how to focus their leadership efforts and achieve Triple Aim results – better health, better care, at lower cost – for the populations they serve. High-impact leadership is required.'

Mindful leadership is high impact because its remit is to refashion the transactional culture thus opening a space for better health and better care. I cannot make claims for lower cost yet given the 'staff cost' of health care, if that resource was effectively led, imagine the consequences!

Footnote

I hope people are excited by leadership and want to become leaders at every level of the organisation. I am more than happy to work with organisations if they need guidance to accomplish this.

c.johns198@btinternet.com

Notes

1. www.brainyquote.com/quotes/quotes/l/laotzu108135.html
2. See Chapter 1 pages 21–23.
3. See Chapter 5.
4. See Pia's narrative (Chapter 8).
5. I met with each ward manager for an hour every four weeks for a minimum of one year.

The MSc Health Care Leadership Programme

The MSc Health Care Leadership programme was established in 2002. It comprises six modules that inform the core narrative dissertation delivered over 28 months. The structure of the programme is outlined in Table A1.1. The programme requires the aspiring leaders to construct a narrative of their reflexive journey towards becoming a leader using significant reflected-on experiences. These narratives are deeply insightful and have evidenced the ideas throughout this book.

The programme is open to all health and social care practitioners.

Community of inquiry

The learning milieu is the community of inquiry, whereby the aspiring leaders are guided to learn through reflections on their experiences of becoming a leader. In this way, the programme is tailor made for each leader, irrespective of role, discipline and experience. The community is a dialogical space where emerging leaders voice and deepen their insights with their guides and peers who are experiencing similar developmental journeys. This dialogue creates a synergistic energy that is greater than working with individual leaders (Johns 2003). What one leader shares, others will also be experiencing, prompting their own reflections.

Hooks (1994: 40) writes:

> Working with a critical pedagogy based on my understanding of Freire's teaching, I enter the classroom with the assumption that we must build 'community' ... I think that a feeling of community creates a sense that there is shared commitment and a common good that binds us ... One way to build community is to recognise the value of each individual voice.

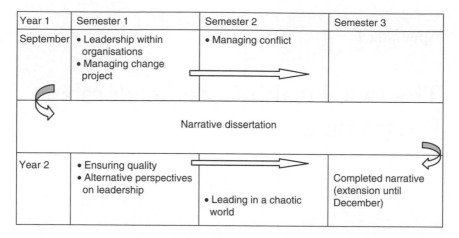

Year 1	Semester 1	Semester 2	Semester 3
September	• Leadership within organisations • Managing change project	• Managing conflict	
	Narrative dissertation		
Year 2	• Ensuring quality • Alternative perspectives on leadership	• Leading in a chaotic world	Completed narrative (extension until December)

Table A1.1 The MSc Health Care Leadership modular programme

The significance of creating community cannot be emphasised enough, simply because it is what the leader must establish within her leadership practice. In other words there is always resonance between learning and practice modes of being.

The community is guided to establish optimum conditions for dialogue and ensure its effective performance. In doing so, the guide is mindful of creating a *liberating structure* that goes against the grain of an instrumental pedagogy and the transactional nature of health care organisations. Torbert (1978) notes that the defining aspect of a liberating structure is opening a negotiated and collaborative space whereby educational processes are congruent and transparent with negotiated desired outcomes. The space is shaped so the emerging leaders can realise their leadership aspirations as a continued thread of meaning through a constant cycle of experimentation and feedback on their actions to realise leadership. The aspiring leader learns to witness and monitor the development of her leadership. Nothing is ever static but always in a dynamic state of disequilibrium. One aspect of a liberating structure is 'social jiujitsu' whereby guides develop the capacity to communicate on two levels. The first level is the language people know and respond to – the language of transactional management. Simultaneously, the guide begins to communicate in a new desirable leadership language that undermines the old language. It is a process of creative transition as the new way of talking takes hold.

For the community to work at its most effective, each member accepts responsibility for their own performance within it and for the community's performance as a whole. This idea of taking responsibility is not easy when people have been socialised to be subordinate. Taking responsibility means 'coming out' as a leader as played out in the community of inquiry. Gathering strength, the aspiring leader then begins to take responsibility for her leadership in practice.

Within the community of inquiry leadership ebbs and flows at appropriate moments – at times active and intense and, at other times, passive, yet ever present, smouldering. Like quiet service, leadership is often subtle, unobtrusive, empathic, intuitive and perceptive. Greenleaf (2002: 35) writes, 'People grow taller when those who lead them empathise and when they are accepted for what they are, even though their performance may be judged critically in terms of what they are capable of doing.'

The community of inquiry is a whole brain space that nurtures and assimilates right and left brain attributes as a praxis: a space where reason and logic meet imagination and creativity. Artists work with the aspiring leaders to move the student leaders beyond conceptual thinking into a greater wholeness. For many of the student leaders this is not easy because the imagination has been trimmed. Paramananda writes (2001: 70/71),

> Of course the sad thing, the tragic thing, is that many of us do get trimmed. We all start off with real heads full of space and imagination, but slowly, somewhere along the path that we call growing up, our heads get trimmed. We become caught up in the doings of this world, the realities of adult life, and we cut down to size.

Cut down to size, the aspiring leaders feel intimidated by the idea of play or feel they are not creative, or can even be creative. They paint and write to create themselves as leaders.

Dialogue is the pattern of verbal communication for leadership. As such, it is the pattern of communication consciously used within the leadership's community of inquiry. It is something appreciated and cultured through action and reflection where other, more dominant patterns of organisational talk that characterise transactional life, are exposed and challenged. Using dialogue transforms the organisation.

The majority of theory is fed into the dialogue as appropriate to inform practice. To maintain the flow of the leadership programme the director of studies guides all modules whilst bringing in experts to inform the leaders around specific topics, for example, quality strategy. All module assignments require action and reflection, leading to the emergence of leadership insight.

A summary of each module is outlined in Table A1.2.

The community of inquiry is a nice idea, yet the university is a potential oppressive force in the way it determines the nature of teaching and

Module	Description	Assignment
Leadership in organisations	Leaders are guided to: • Explore the idea of leadership and to construct a personal vision of leadership drawing on contemporary leadership literature • Analyse the organisational culture of their workplace • Appreciate the creative tension between transformational leadership and the transactional organisation and position self within that tension • Maintain a reflective journal and contribute these experiences to the community of inquiry • Understand that the key role of leadership is to create and sustain the learning organisation (Senge 1990) • Review and develop existing visions for practice (as a key role of leadership) • Appreciate the barriers to rational change (Fay 1987): power, tradition and embodiment Reflect on experiences of leadership written in journals and shared within group-guided reflection seminars	Reflect on a recent experience that reveals something about becoming a leader and the constraints of achieving this within the organisation.
Positive conflict resolution	Leaders are guided to: • Reflect on experiences of conflict within their everyday practice within group-guided reflection seminars • Position self within styles of responding to conflict situations from the perspective of leadership (using Thomas and Kilmann conflict management grid) • Consider the influence of gender in conflict (linked to power, tradition and embodiment) • Explore the ethical nature of practice and ethical decision-making in resolving dilemmas and conflict • Explore and develop the nature of empowerment and assertiveness • Understand the demands of everyday practice on self boundaries and ways these demands can be responded to in terms of shared success View conflict as a positive phenomenon within the learning organisation	Reflect on at least two situations of conflict and one's mode of response; explore the tension between one's actual mode of response and one's desired mode in tune with leadership values.

(Continued)

Leading change	Leaders are guided to: • Lead self as a leader and as a change agent • Lead a change project through design, implementation and evaluation • Review their lived response to resistance • Reflect on their change leadership through the lens of diverse change theories to inform their learning and possibilities for responding to change in other ways • Write a project management report applying a formal project management tool Work collaboratively as a group to organise a profitable change conference and give a conference paper (subsequently edited within conference proceedings)	Design, implement and lead a change project. Write a project report suitable for organisational review with separate chapters on managing resistance and insights gained in leading change.
Ensuring quality	Leaders are guided to: • Appreciate the nature of clinical governance and the ways in which it works within their own organisations – is it effective? • Consider what is best practice? How might it be known? • Develop the potential of using clinical audit in their practice (through creating a clinical audit environment within seminars using leaders' own reflections on realising best practice) • Critically review the potential for establishing effective clinical supervision within practice • Develop and lead a quality project linked into clinical governance, including evaluation • Write a quality project report on the results Work collaboratively as a group to organise a profitable quality conference and give a conference paper (subsequently edited within conference proceedings)	Design, implement and lead a quality project. Write a report for organisational review.
Alternative perspectives on leadership	Leaders are guided to: • Shadow and reflect on the leadership of another leader within their organisation • Consider the nature of group dynamics • Review frameworks of leadership and select appropriate frameworks to reflect on the leader's leadership Contrast results with the leaders' own emerging leadership	Write an account of shadowing a leader using appropriate reflective frameworks of leadership and contrast with your own emerging leadership.

(Continued)

181

Module	Description	Assignment
Leading in a chaotic world	Leaders are guided to: • Contrast a chaos view of the world with the (generally prevailing) Newtonian view and the way these views link with organisation culture and leadership • Reflect on feedback loops through the leaders' own experiences and the significance of feedback loops in holding the creative edge within the learning organisation • Reflect on appreciating the significance of strange attractors, the butterfly effect and patterning within leadership experiences Loosen the bindings of organisational anxiety in order to explore the potential of a chaotic view of the world	A reflective account on the impact of chaos theory on your leadership.

Table A1.2 Summary of taught modules

learning within normative parameters. I was inspired by Freire's ideas on a liberating pedagogy. He writes (1972: 68),

> *The starting point for organizing the programme content of education or political action must be the present, existential, concrete situation, reflecting the aspirations of the people. Utilizing certain basic contradictions, we must pose this existential, concrete, present situation to the people as a problem which challenges them and requires a response – not just at the intellectual level, but at the level of action. We must never merely discourse on the present situation, must never provide the people with programmes which have little or nothing to do with their preoccupations, doubts, hopes and fears – programmes which at times in fact increase the fears of the oppressed consciousness. It is not our role to speak to the people about our own view, not to attempt to impose that view on them, but rather to dialogue with the people about their view and ours.*

Reflection

Leaders are required to reflect on and share experiences of being and becoming a leader within the community of inquiry that meets for one day every two weeks throughout the programme. Reflection is learning through one's everyday lived experience towards realising one's vision of leadership as a lived reality. Learning is reflected through insights, which, by their very nature, change the way the leader perceives and responds to the world, within a reflexive spiral of becoming as evidenced within the narrative. The word 'reflexive' captures the sense of *looking back* to see self emerging as a leader through a series of reflected-on experiences where one experience builds on previous ones. It is a chain, where each link of the chain is informed by the previous one (Dewey 1933).

Schön (1983, 1987) made a distinction between reflection-on-experience and reflection-in-action. Reflection-in-action is posited as a type of problem solving in the midst of doing something. The problem is reframed, which may involve thinking differently, so the activity can continue. He also proposed a radical shift in the epistemology of professional practice. He recognised that the sort of knowing most valuable for professionals was practical knowing learnt through reflection. He argued that most of the problems that faced professionals were complex and indeterminate and defied any rule following – what he termed *the swampy lowlands*. As such, it makes sense to reflect on those experiences in order to learn through them and develop ways such problems might be best solved, drawing on any relevant theory or research to inform this process.

Through reflection, the leaders learn to hold creative tension – the tension between a vision of leadership, itself a moveable feast, and an understanding of their current reality. The aim is to understand this tension and work towards resolving it in order to live one's vision of leadership as a lived reality. The leader comes to appreciate that the factors that constrain their realisation of leadership are deeply rooted in themselves and within organisational culture. Understanding these factors, grounded in issues of authority, tradition and embodiment (Fay 1987), helps to disentangle the leader from the influence of them. However, these factors are deeply embodied within the leader and reinforced daily within normal patterns of relating. This is particularly true for nurses who have been socialised to be subordinate, resulting in low self-esteem and low confidence. Yet these constraints are not real. One's understanding of current reality can be distorted by a false perception of self and events (Lather 1993).

Model for structured reflection

To facilitate reflection I constructed the model for structured reflection (MSR) (Figure A1.1). It consists of a sequential cues designed to systematically structure self-inquiry.[1] The MSR was initially constructed in 1990 through analysing the pattern of questions used in guiding nurses to learn through experience and framed within the grounded theory paradigm model (Johns 2013). Since then, the MSR has been constantly tested and

Reflective cue
Bring the mind home
Focus on a description of an experience that seems significant in some way (usually written in a journal)
What particular issues seem significant to pay attention to?
How were others feeling and why did they feel that way?
How was I feeling and what made me feel that way?
What was I trying to achieve and was I effective?
What were the consequences of my actions on the patient, others and myself?
What knowledge informed or might have informed me?
How does this situation connect with previous experiences?
To what extent did I act for the best and in tune with my (leadership) values?
What factors influence the way I was/am feeling, thinking and responding to this situation?
What are my underlying assumptions that govern my practice, what is the basis for these assumptions and how do I need to shift them in order to realise more effective practice?
How do my assumptions that govern my practice need to shift in order to realise my vision of self?
How might I reframe the situation and respond more effectively given this situation again?
What would be the consequences of alternative actions for the patient, others and myself?
What factors might constrain me from responding in new ways?
How do I NOW feel about this experience?
Am I more able to support myself and others better as a consequence?
What insights do I draw from this experience?

Figure A1.1 The model for structured reflection (Edition 16)

refined. The cues are not intended to be prescriptive; they are heuristics, a means towards gaining insights. Over time, with practice, the aspiring leader internalises and uses the cues naturally both to reflect on her practice and more significantly within practice itself. To reiterate, the disciplined approach to reflection develops self-awareness and ultimately mindfulness – the ability to hold creative tension moment by moment.

Bringing the mind home brings the leaders into a mindful space prior to reflection and indeed before all action. Then the mind is not distracted and able to focus with undivided attention. This is achieved using breathing techniques, taking a meditation posture.

Through description aspiring leaders learn to pay attention to experience. It may appear mundane, yet every experience, when we pay attention to it, is significant. When the leader returns to practice, she is more aware of herself and those things she has paid attention to and reflected on. In this way mindfulness is cultivated. Imagine the power and value of such practice day after day.

Della writes: From the very first day I kept a reflective journal to capture the essence of my emerging leadership journey. This enabled me to articulate memories and events and begin to interpret some of my articulation in a private space; a space where I could tell myself stories and liberate my voice as a woman and as a practitioner, by choosing words that reflected my own personal values as I uttered them in my text. My journaling permitted me to be creative and allowed me to immerse self into a space that was mine, allowing me to live leadership as a reality.

Feelings

The first reflective cues are concerned with feelings, acknowledging the significance that feelings have for decision practice and action (Callahan 1988). Indeed, it is our feelings that often draw our attention to experience, something unsettling perhaps that disturbs sleep. The mindful leader is aware that feelings may interfere with reason, yet, as Callahan argues, 'the emotions and reason should be mutually correcting' (9). Senge (1990) considers that the aspiring leader will need to work through emotional tension in order to see reality more clearly, suggesting that strong emotions distort perception of reality. In doing so, emotional tension can be converted into positive energy for taking action towards resolving creative tension.

It helps the aspiring leader to pay attention and release her feelings through the words we write, especially when those feelings are trapped. Writing a story is cathartic and healing (De Salvo 1999). Anxiety is harmful to the body, especially anxiety that is not resolved. The fight–flight response is no longer socially acceptable – we simply can't hit people or walk out of the unit. So people often do not have an outlet for this destructive energy. Proverbs like 'kicking the dog' come to mind. The reflective effort is to accept and understand this anxiety so it can be converted into positive energy for resolving causes of anxiety. Feelings are very influential in determining responses to situations and hence it is vital for the leaders to acknowledge their feelings and understand their nature.

> Sam writes: Hooks (1990: 34) suggests that human actions are determined and shaped by the larger circumstances within which those individuals find themselves. My inner turmoil appears a direct result of the larger circumstance. Chris helps me release my emotional tension. A necessary cathartic release before I can hold creative tension and consider ways to move into the right place to realise my vision as a practice educator effectively. I can begin to unravel the organisational complexity for what it is.

Through reflecting on how others were feeling within the particular situation, the leader cultivates the quality of empathic inquiry (Cope 2001) – the quality of tuning into the other person and understanding the other's perspective. Understanding how the other person is feeling is vital in terms of responding to the other person(s) in ways congruent with transformational leadership. Leaders recognise feelings and use catharsis to enable others to appropriately express their feelings and create the conditions for creative tension, dialogue and positive conflict resolution. The leaders also recognise their own feelings. Feelings such as guilt, anger, anxiety, frustration and impatience lead to unskilful action. As such, reflection always intends to cultivate positive emotions leading to a healthy sympathetic resonance in response to others, what is termed poise or emotional intelligence – the ability to know and manage self.

What was I trying to achieve?

All action is purposeful, governed by a vision of what the person seeks to achieve. This may be a broad picture like a vision statement or an objective to be realised within the particular situation.

Was I effective?

The *craft* of leadership is reflected in the performance of leadership. Craft has four movements:

1. Appreciating the particular situation. The situation is seen clearly for what it is. It involves framing the particular situation within the bigger

picture and seeing the relationship between things and how attitudes and systems impact upon it.

2. Making decisions as to *how best* to respond in terms of what is hoped to be achieved. *How best* reflects both empirical and ethical influences – reflecting that the leader is both widely informed and deeply concerned to do the right thing. Leadership is conscience to act with integrity.

3. The leader is concerned with responding with appropriate skilled and moral action to help others meet their needs and enable growth.

4. Gaining feedback to ensure that actions lead to desired outcomes and that systems are adequate to support practice. Feedback might involve audit and debriefing systems to ensure that every situation is a learning opportunity and that nothing is taken for granted.

Whilst these movements have a logical sequence, they are in dynamic flow. The leader may not even be aware of these movements in response. She may have an intuitive *feel* for the patterns of what is unfolding. Wheatley (1999: 126) suggests a reflective posture helps us see and appreciate pattern.

> *To see patterns, we have to step back from the problem and gain perspective. Shapes are not discerned from close range. They require distance and time to show themselves. Pattern recognition requires that we sit together reflectively and patiently. I say patiently not just because patterns take time to form, but because we are trying to see the world differently and there are many years of blindness to overcome.*

As I shall develop in subsequent cues, the way the leader responds is further influenced by:

- The ethical – acting for the best in terms of the right thing to do
- The empirical – acting in accordance with evidence of best practice
- The personal – the influence of values, assumptions, past experience, stress, mental models, confidence, assertiveness and suchlike

What were the consequences of my actions for self and others?

The old adage – actions have consequences. This cue prompts the leader to consider the consequences of her actions beyond their more obvious impact. What are or might be the hidden and longer-term consequences of actions? This is also a moral issue concerned with creating better worlds for people. All too often, the reactive and short-term fix creates problems for the future. By considering consequences of actions, the leader develops practical wisdom: the ability to be mindful in weighing up consequences before acting – the antidote for the reactive transactional culture. Remember Nelson Mandela's words: 'A good head and a good heart are always a formidable combination'. In other words, leaders are both wise and compassionate and able to balance heart with mind. The community of inquiry resembles the Native American powwow whereby we sit around and deeply reflect on issues, dispelling strong emotional influences, until we know how best to respond within any particular situation.

Informed by knowledge

The cue 'What knowledge informed or might have informed me?' challenges the leader to critique and assimilate any ideas from whatever source to inform their practice related to the particular experience. All ideas are viewed sceptically for their value and authority to inform the particular situation. Such knowing can never be taken on face value or applied mindlessly because every human–human encounter is unique and previous ways of knowing can never be routinely applied. This requires research appreciation skills of critiquing often complex research papers for their authority to inform. Thus the leader is always an *informed* leader, addressing the dominant health care agenda of evidence-based practice. In truth, there is little evidence to inform much of what Schön (1983, 1987) describes as *the swampy lowlands* of clinical practice that are complex and indeterminate without prescribed answers. Indeed, as the narratives portray, the leader learns to find her way through reflection.

Looking back

The cue 'How does this situation connect with previous experiences?' acknowledges the impact of past experience on decision-making. Leaders, as with all practitioners, get locked into patterns of thinking and habitual practice that may not be congruent with effective leadership. As such, leaders liberate themselves from the tyranny of learnt patterns and the status quo in order to make decisions. The cue challenges the way practitioners tend to make decisions based on three generally unreflective criteria:

- What they know and have used before
- What they are comfortable with
- What has worked previously

Through reflection these criteria are examined and considered for their influence on what is happening now.

The moral maze

Transformational leadership is moral seeking to lift people to higher levels of morality (Burns, 1978). Leadership is always striving to create better worlds for staff and patients within health care. Any other type of leadership would be perverse or, in fact, could not be described as leadership. In considering the cue *'To what extent did I act for the best and in tune with my (leadership) values?'*, the leader must consider the nature of *for the best*. This necessitates an understanding of key ethical principles and the way these might guide decision-making and action. The leader is often faced with a dilemma – should I do this or should I do that? Inevitably other people are involved who may view the situation differently. To help resolve ethical dilemmas I constructed the 'ethical map' (Figure A1.2). The map guides the leader to consider the dilemma from the different perspectives of all people involved. This encourages an empathic understanding, challenging the leader's own partial view of the situation that helps her loosen any emotional attachment to her own perspective. Only when these different perspectives are mutually understood is resolution possible. When people are attached to their partial views they do not listen to other perspectives. The leader then considers the way ethical principles inform the situation, notably autonomy, beneficence, non-malevolence and utilitarianism. There is always tension

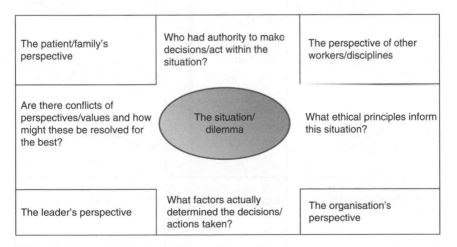

Figure A1.2 Ethical mapping
Source: Adapted from Johns 1999, 2009

within autonomy – the right for self-determination, working within organisations where patterns of authority determine the scope of autonomy. Similarly there is always a tension of autonomy between patients, families and health care practitioners in determining decision-making. There is always tension with finite resources – how should resources best be allocated – leading to issues of time and priorities.

Appreciating the different perspectives, ethical principles and patterns of authority is helpful for resolving any conflict, even though decisions are often made by those with greater authority irrespective of whether it is the best decision or not. However, the leader, acting with integrity according to her leadership values, ensures her voice is clearly listened to.

Influencing factors

The way the leader responds in any situation is influenced by a number of factors. As such, the cue 'What factors are influencing the way I was/ am thinking, feeling and responding to this situation?' has great breadth and depth. These influences are reflected in the Influences grid (Figure A1.3).

Conforming to 'normal practice/ habit'? Past experiences?	Expectations from others as to how I should act?	Particular attitudes/prejudice? Need to be valued?
Limited skills/discomfort/ confidence to act in new ways?		Fear of sanction? Anxiety about ensuing conflict? Need to be in control?
Emotional entanglement/over-identification?	What factors influence my decision-making and actions?	Misplaced concern – loyalty to colleagues versus loyalty to patient?
Personal stuff/baggage? Deeper psyche factors?		Knowledge to act in specific ways?
Wrapped up in self-concern? Pity? Stressed? Guilt? Frustration? Other feelings?	Expectations from self about 'how I should act'	Acting for the good? Time/priorities?

Figure A1.3 Influences grid

I have included *past experiences* and *acting for the good* from the previous cues in order to offer a more comprehensive grid.

The grid is developed around the fundamental tension between expectations of self and expectations from others, influenced by diverse factors that have their roots in the barriers to rational change – embodiment, force and tradition (Fay 1987). Coming to perceive these factors enables the leader to gain an understanding of their current reality – necessary for holding creative tension. All the factors influence the way the leader perceives and responds to practice to varying extent, yet it is not easy for leaders to perceive these forces woven, as they are, deep within self and within the fabric of normal culture. Take for example the way 'fear of sanction' will force people into compliance and subordination. I expect every reader appreciates the message 'Keep your head down or otherwise it will be blown off'. Such is the nature of the transactional organisation layered through its power structures that is intolerant to criticism from its own members. 'If you give them an inch they'll take a mile' – such is the risk of allowing people to voice.

Exploring these factors can be unsettling because they disturb the leader's learnt patterns of mental models that govern self. Constructing new patterns of mental models congruent with desired leadership is also unsettling, as it naturally disrupts normal patters of relationships with others.

Trail:

1. Consider each person's perspective commencing with your own particular perspective. Be aware of your partiality. Draw on your empathy to really appreciate the other person's perspective.
2. Consider what ethical principles might usefully inform the 'best' decision-making – significantly autonomy, beneficence, non-malevolence and utilitarianism.
3. Identify and understand any conflict that exists between perspectives and how this might be 'ethically' resolved for the best.
4. Consider who has authority to make decisions and the process of decision-making.
5. Reflect on the way the decision was actually made and what can be learnt from this in terms of future decision-making and professional relationships.

What are my underlying assumptions that govern my practice and what is the basis for these assumptions?
How do my assumptions that govern my practice need to shift in order to realise my vision of self?

The way we practise is governed by the assumptions we hold. These assumptions are embodied and generally taken for granted. In other words they are normal for us and for others working within specific environments. On one level, such assumptions may seem implicit within the influences grid, but on another level it moves insights gained from the influences grid into a deeper appreciation of self. Introducing the cue opens a space to formally summarise ideas generated by the influences grid and then to ask 'What is the basis for these assumptions?' – given that we need to appreciate them in order to shift them into line with our vision of becoming a leader.

Looking forward

The looking forward cues are designed to guide the leader to anticipate how he or she might respond more effectively given the same situation. Of course such consideration doesn't determine how the leader will actually respond. The cue 'What factors might constrain me from responding in new ways?' is intended to keep the options grounded in possibility rather than fantasy. Generating options and their consequences opens up the leader's imagination and perception to see the possibilities of responding in more effective ways. It challenges normative ways of thinking about situations and to think outside the box – the antidote for unreflective action. These options are like seeds planted in the mind to germinate and bloom in subsequent experience as appropriate. They prepare the leader to anticipate new situations.

How do I NOW feel?

Without doubt, practice in health care is both emotional and stressful, steeped as it is in human suffering and conflict through working in toxic transactional environments. Reflection lifts this emotional tension to the surface where it can be resolved. Resolution converts negative energy into positive energy for the leader to act on her insights. The cue helps promote self-esteem and perseverance, acknowledging that things are not necessarily easy to shift quickly.

Supporting self and others

Linked to the previous cue, it is a revelation to appreciate just how isolated many leaders feel and the high level of strain they experience (Johns 2003). Often reflection reveals the poorly developed support systems for leaders within practice and their own lack of self-care. The transformational leader seeks to establish mutually supportive relationships with staff based on thick trust, to deal with emotional tension that drains their energy and can be demoralising when emotional tension is unremitting.

Gaining insights

Having scanned the MSR cues along the reflective spiral, the aspiring leader pulls together the threads of information revealed through the reflective cues to consider what *tentative* insights she has gained. By *tentative* I mean they are held loosely or warrant deeper scrutiny through subsequent dialogical movements. Insights are changed perspectives of self. They are not simply ideas. Neither do they necessarily emerge rationally. More often they are moments of insight as if something clicks. Ah-ha! As such, they are not always easily articulated or perhaps so subtle that the student leader is not consciously aware of the insight. Such insights are only revealed through subsequent experience and reflection. To gain insight, the leader needs to dwell on the text and be open to possibilities of what the text might reveal.

Okri (1997: 22) captures this quest: 'Hold them. Look at them. Play with them. See where they lead. Every perception or possibility has its own life-span: some have short lives, others keep on growing, and many are open to infusions of greater life'.

This is an imaginative process. Tufnell and Crickmay (2004: 119) note, 'Imagination is not a separate faculty – rather it engages all parts of our mind and intelligence – fusing or bringing together often surprising aspects of what we know or feel, imagination expands our seeing.'

Reflection nurtures the creative, imaginative, perceptive, intuitive and empathic qualities of being – all qualities essential for effective leadership – blended with reason in perfect balance. The aspiring leader learns to dwell patiently on her text. The quality of patience is like watching a washing machine. With every cycle of the wash another insight is thrown out. Wisdom is not rushed. Insights can be framed within the framing perspectives, which offer a systematic approach to review learning through reflection (Figure A1.4). Philosophical and role framing are fundamental perspectives because all practice is value driven and governed by role. Theoretical framing has been touched on with the cue '*What knowledge informed or might have informed me?*'.

Reality perspective framing gets to the heart of creative tension in becoming a leader. Problem framing is inspired by Schön's idea of reflection in action, the ability to pause within practice and reframe the situation in

Framing perspective	How has this experience enabled me to:
• Philosophical framing	confront and clarify my beliefs and values that constitute desirable clinical and leadership practice?
• Role framing	clarify my role boundaries and authority within my role, and my power relationships with others?
• Theoretical framing	identify and critically assimilate into personal knowing relevant theory and research to inform or frame my knowing in practice?
• Reality perspective framing	understand the barrier of reality (systems/ mental models/embodiment/power/tradition) that constrains my practice as a leader whilst enabling me to become empowered to act in more congruent ways as a leader?
• Problem framing	focus problem identification and resolution within the particular experience?
• Temporal framing	draw patterns with past experiences whilst anticipating how I might respond in similar situations in new, more effective, ways?
• Parallel process framing	make connections between learning processes within guided reflection and my practice as a leader? For example, dialogue within the community of learning and dialogue within my practice.
• Developmental framing	monitor my leadership development in tune with my vision from a whole perspective?

Figure A1.4 Framing perspectives

order to move on with it. Temporal framing links the present with the past by acknowledging the way the past influences the present whilst anticipating how the leader may respond differently, more effectively perhaps, in future similar situations. It draws together the looking back and looking MSR cues. Parallel process framing is concerned with the transfer of learning between guided reflection and leadership practice. Developmental framing refers to the reflexive framing of leadership emergence using appropriate leadership frameworks, for example the 'being available' template.

Gayle, a modern matron, writes: Had I fully comprehended the nature of the leadership programme I may not have proceeded with the course. The reflective process has been integral to the whole programme. Reflection may have not been what I wanted, but I believe it's what I needed. By gaining insights into the interpersonal dynamics of my own behaviour I recognise and realise aspects of myself or patterns of behaviour that I was unaware of. Certain parts of the process have been self-revelatory. The ongoing process has changed who I am, how I think and how I behave. The effects are subtle, but I believe significant. I feel better able to challenge the transactional culture by understanding my role within it.

Appendix 2

Narrative Construction

Since 2002, aspiring leaders on the MSc Health Care Leadership programme have written more than eighty narratives. These narratives reveal the leaders' journeys of becoming a leader within transactional health care organisations. The methodology is 'reflexive narrative' – a journey of self-inquiry and transformation towards realising one's vision of leadership as a lived reality (Johns 2010). This approach to research offers a meaningful and practical approach to practitioner research that is deeply compelling in its authenticity and its impact on enabling leadership.

Reflexive narratives are constructed from stories (reflections on experiences) linked reflexively together to vividly portray the emergence of leadership (the plot) and an understanding of those forces that have constrained such emergence, for example, patterns of organisational relationships that structure and govern everyday life. This is particularly apposite in reflexive narrative that seeks not merely to understand those relationships but to transform them towards becoming a mindful leader.

Narratives have become significant within health care research. Narratives of illness (Frank 2002) reflect on the experience and meaning of illness. The works of such theorists such as Clandinin and Connelly (2000) and Mattingley (1998), amongst others, have brought narrative research, with its roots in ethnography, into the mainstream, usually through researching other peoples' stories. Self-inquiry, for example as auto-ethnography (Bochner and Ellis 2002), opens the path for clinicians to research self, as exemplified in my own approach with its emphasis on not just understanding self but transforming self (Johns 2010, 2013). This approach blends guided reflection, narrative, critical social science, hermeneutics and more esoteric influences such as feminism, Native American lore and Buddhism into a cohesive process.

Six dialogical movements

Narrative is constructed through six dialogical movements within the hermeneutic circle (Figure A2.1). The hermeneutic circle is the dialogue between the whole of one's understanding (what is in the circle) and the new meanings or insights emerging from reflection. This leads to a reflexive deepening of wholeness of being a leader. The six movements are in constant flow.

First dialogical movement

The first movement is to write a story as a rich description of an experience that in someway seems significant in being a leader. It is significant to write the story because the process of writing opens the perceptual mind. It focuses the student leader to pay attention and draw on all her senses.

Writing is a creative and imaginative process. Loori (2004: 90) writes:

> In the creative process, as long as the energy is strong, the process continues. It may take minutes or hours. As long as you feel chi peaking and flowing, let it run its course. It's important to allow this flow and expression, without attempting to edit what is happening, without trying to name, judge, analyse, or understand it. The time for editing is later. The time for uninhibited flow of expression is now.

The writer strives to recall the essence of any experience as accurately as possible. However, they are cognisant of the natural tension between a mimetic stance that seeks to accurately recall the detail of the experience and an anti-mimetic stance that acknowledges that is not possible or even desirable (Mattingley 1998). At first, the aspiring leaders tend to reflect on experiences that are negative in nature. This is natural because these are the experiences that most come to mind. These types of experiences are often emotional and expose the starkness of tension between vision and reality.

Karen writes: I chose not to take these two experiences to guided reflection because they were positive. I felt no pressing need to dig deeper with a guide. Maybe I am still in the place whereby I am only able to reflect deeply on issues that are negative and centred around my own trauma.

1.	Dialogue with self to write a rich descriptive story of a particular significant experience (story text)
2.	Dialogue with the story text, as an objective and disciplined process using a model of reflection to gain insight (reflective text)
3.	Dialogue between the text and relevant sources of knowing in order to frame insights within the wider community of knowing
4.	Dialogue between the text's author and guides and peers within the community of learning to check out and deepen insights
5.	Dialogue with the emerging text to weave the pattern of insights into a coherent and reflexive narrative (narrative text)
6.	Dialogue with others (through published text, performance and play) towards consensus and social action (consensual text)

Figure A2.1 John's (2010) six dialogical movements

> Della writes: From the very first day I kept a reflective journal to capture the essence of my emerging leadership journey. This enabled me to articulate memories and events and begin to interpret some of my articulation in a private space; a space where I could tell self stories and liberate my voice as a woman and as a practitioner, by choosing words that reflected my own personal values as I uttered them in my text. My journaling permitted me to be creative and allowed me to immerse self into a space that was mine, allowing me to live leadership as a reality.

The guide encourages leaders to pay attention to positive experiences as well as negative experiences to give positive feedback of achievement and counter the frustration of constant negative experiences.

> Luke writes: The journal entries opened my mind to see the gap between my values and my actual clinical practice. Insights from these diary entries occurred because an issue had been bubbling just beneath the surface for some time. From these insights, potent realisations of repetitive behavioural patterns arose, from which I could begin the journey of personal transformation. However, keeping a journal is like having a friend who is a little too honest about you, thus if we do hear the truth we may turn hastily away. James (2003) wrote that we avoid depression or fear by insulating ourselves in illusions. Thus my journal entries may occasionally have pre-empted the pain they could cause;

(Continued)

therefore there is the danger that painful truths are hidden in softness and sugar. Another limitation of journal writing is the temptation to fabricate, minimise or silence myself because of fear of giving myself away to the reader. The narratives may be governed by expectations about being seen as 'normal' or to only include 'good' stories (Aranda and Street 2001). This loss of truthfulness may impoverish learning by choosing order and structure due to fear of being seen as 'different'.

Second dialogical movement

Having written a description of an experience, the leader stands back from the text to view it more objectively in order to reflect on it towards gaining insight. This facilitates reflection. Both a model of structured reflection (Figure A1.1) and guidance are necessary to explore the breadth and depth of reflection and to counter the leaders' partial perception of self.

Third dialogical movement

Holding tentative insights, leaders dialogue with the wider community of knowing to develop their insights. In this way, the leader deepens her ability to use information creatively to inform her practice and develop rationale for her actions. This is significant within a transactional health care organisation that values objective information on which to base its decisions. Story illuminates the cold facts of theory and research into something real and personal. Story is often viewed pejoratively as anecdote and dismissed. Perhaps the cold face of the transactional prefers the impersonal as a way of avoiding the truth of situations as lived.

Fourth dialogical movement

The aspiring leaders share their experiences and insights within the community of inquiry with peers and guides. Here, insights are challenged, guiding the leader to see beyond their own partial horizons. In this way insights are co-created and deepened.

Fifth dialogical movement

The leaders weave together the narrative of realising their leadership using a series of significant experiences that reflexively plot and evidence the emergence and transformation of self as a leader. Transformation can be marked by utilising leadership frameworks indicative of the leader's vision as evidenced within the narratives. This strengthens narrative form and coherence. The idea of coherence challenges the leader to consider why someone would believe the narrative. What makes it authentic and convincing? Weaving narrative is creative whereby the leaders develop their own style of narrative, utilising poetry, art, even play style that reflects synergy between the yin and yang, the masculine and feminine and the right and left brain.

Sixth dialogical movement

The narrative opens a dialogical space to engage with an audience.

Background

In constructing the narrative background, the leader positions herself in context of her leadership journey to enable readers to gain a perspective of who she is. This is achieved utilising Heidegger's (1962) concept of fore-structure. This has three aspects: fore-having, fore-sight, and fore-conception.

Fore-having – the leader reviews her life history identifying defining experiences that seem to influence how she sees and responds to the world and how she comes to be the person she is today. Writing the background enables the leader to see the significance of past experiences and their impact on becoming a leader. Through reviewing the past, the leaders can make sense of the attitudes, emotions and assumptions they hold about themselves and their practice. These experiences often stem back to childhood as the leaders come to appreciate such influences on their leadership behaviour.

Fore-sight – the leader positions self in context of her current perspectives, roles, organisation, and suchlike. It sets out the nature of the leader's current practice and role, responsibilities and relationships, and current issues that feel significant in some way.

Fore-conception – the leader sets out her preliminary vision of leadership literature and her projections of what she expects the journey will be like – a kind of anticipation that may be realistic or delusional reflecting the leader's personality, for example, are they optimistic or pessimistic? There is clearly a temporal link between the past and the future, between fore-having and fore-conception.

Notes

1. See Johns (2014) for a comprehensive appreciation of reflection.

References

Adamson, E., King, L., Moody, J. and Waugh, A. (2009) Developing a nursing education project in partnership: Leadership in compassionate care. *Nursing Times*, 105(35): 23–6.

Alfano, G. (1971) Healing or caretaking – Which will it be? *Nursing Clinics of North America*, 6(2): 273–80.

Alimo-Metcalfe, B. (2002) Confounding myths around leadership. *Community Practitioner*, 75(12): 450.

Aranda, S. and Street, A. (2001) From individual to group: Use of narratives in a participatory research process. *Journal of Advanced Nursing*, 33(6): 791–7.

Argyris, C. (1982) *Reasoning, learning and action: Individual and organisational*. Jossey Bass, San Francisco, CA.

Ashman, M., Read, S., Savage, J. and Scott, C. (2006) Outcomes of modern matron implementation: Trust nursing directors' perceptions and case study findings. *Clinical Effectiveness in Nursing*, 9(supplement 1): 44–52.

Badaracco, J. (2002) *Leading quietly*. Harvard Business School Press, Boston, MA.

Barber, P. (1993) Developing the 'person' of the professional carer. In Hinchliff, S., Norman, S. and Schober, J. (Eds) *Nursing practice and health care* (2nd edition). Edward Arnold, London, pp. 344–73.

Barker, A. M. and Young, C. (1994) Transformational leadership: The feminist connection in post-modern organizations. *Holistic Nursing Practice*, 9(1): 16–25.

Bass, B. (1985) *Leadership and performance beyond expectations*. Free Press, New York.

Bass, B. (1990) From transactional to transformational leadership: Learning to share the vision. *Organizational Dynamics*, Winter: 19–31.

Beck, C. Y. (1997) *Everyday Zen*. Thorsons, London.

Belenky, M., Clinchy, B., Goldberger, N. and Tarule, J. (1986) *Women's ways of knowing: The development of self, voice and mind*. Basic Books, New York.

Bennett, J. and Robinson, A. (2003) Developing leadership capacity in community nursing: Meeting the challenge. *Journal of Community Nursing*, 17(1): 22–4.

Bennis, W., Benne, K. D. and Chin, R. (1984) *The planning of change* (4th edition). Holt, Rinehart & Winston, Fort Worth, TX.

Bennis, W. and Nanus, B. (1985) *Leadership: The strategies for taking charge*. John Wiley & Sons, New York.

Berne, E. (1961) *Transactional analysis in psychotherapy*. Grove Press, New York.

Berne, E. (1964) *Games people play*. Penguin Books, London.

Bochner, A. and Ellis, C. (2002) *Ethnographically speaking*. AltaMira Press, Walnut Creek, CA.

Bohm, D. (1996) *On dialogue* (ed. L. Nichol). Routledge, London.

Bolman, L. and Deal, T. (1995) *Leading with soul*. Jossey-Bass, San Francisco, CA.

Boyd, D. (1996) *Rolling thunder*. Delta, New York.

Burnes, B. (1990) *Managing change: A strategic approach to organisational development in renewal*. Pitman, London.

Burns, J. M. (1978) *Leadership*. Harper & Row, New York.

Callahan, S (1988) The role of emotion in ethical decision making. *Hastings Center Report*, 18: 9–14.

Cassidy, V. and Koroll, C. (1994) Ethical aspects of transformational leadership. *Holistic Nursing Practice*, 9: 41–7.

Cavanagh, S. (1991) The conflict management style of staff nurses and managers. *Journal of Advanced Nursing*, 16: 1254–60.

Chambers, N. (2002) Nursing leadership: The time has come to just do it. *Journal of Nursing Management*, 10: 127–8.

Chambers, N. (2005) *Oxford English dictionary* (3rd edition). Oxford University Press, Oxford.

Cixous, H. (1999) *The third body*. Hydra Books, North Western University Press, Evanston, IL.

Clandinin, D. and Connelly, F. (2000) *Narrative inquiry: Experience and story in qualitative research*. Jossey-Bass, San Francisco, CA.

Collins, J. (2001) *Good to great*. Random House Business Books, London.

Cook, M. (2001) The attributes of effective clinical nurse leaders. *Nursing Standard*, 15(35): 33–6.

Cope, M. (2001) *Lead yourself: Who's steering your boat?* Momentum Books, London.

Copnell, B. (1997) Understanding change in clinical nursing practice. *Nursing Inquiry*, 5: 2–10.

Cottrell, S. (1999) *Some current beliefs in the NHS and some consequences for implementing clinical supervision*. Excerpt from conference address. (Online). Available from http://www.clinical-supervision.com (Accessed 18 March 2005).

Covey, S. R. (2002) 'Foreword'. In Greenleaf, Robert *Servant leadership: A journey into the nature of legitimate power and greatness* (25th anniversary edition). Paulist Press, New York/Mahwah, NJ.

Craig, J. and Smyth, R. (2002) *The evidence-based practice manual for nurses*. Churchill Livingstone, Edinburgh.

Critchley, D. (2001) Developing leaders: Making the best use of national leadership programmes. *Nursing Management*, 8(6): 32–3.

Crowe, S. A. (1999) *Since strangling isn't an option*. Berkley Publishing Group, New York.

Cunningham, G. and Kitson, A. (2000) An evaluation of the RCN clinical leadership programme. *Nursing Standard*, 15(13): 34–40.

Davies, C. (1995) *Gender and the professional predicament in nursing*. Open University Press, Buckingham.

Dealey, C., Moss, H., Marshall, J. and Elcoat, C. (2007) Auditing the impact of implementing the modern matron role in an acute teaching trust. *Journal of Nursing Management*, 15(1): 22–33.

Department of Health and Social Security (1986) *Neighbourhood nursing – A focus for care* [Cumberlege Report]. HMSO, London.

Department of Health (1997) *The new NHS: Modern and dependable*. HMSO, London.

Department of Health (1998) *A first class service*. HMSO, London.

Department of Health (1999) *Making a difference: Strengthening the nursing, midwifery and health visiting contribution to health and health care*. HMSO, London.

Department of Health (2001b) *Nearly 2000 modern matrons in the NHS – Two years early*. HMSO, London.

Department of Health (2002a) *Liberating the talents*. HMSO, London.

Department of Health (2002b) *Getting ahead of the curve: A strategy for combating infectious diseases.* HMSO, London.

Department of Health (2003) *Modern matrons – Improving the patient experience.* HMSO, London.

Department of Health (2004a) *Matron's charter: An action plan for cleaner hospitals.* HMSO, London.

Department of Health (2004b) *Choosing health – Making healthy choices easier.* HMSO, London.

Department of Health (2008) *High quality care for all: NHS next stage review final report* [Lord Darzi report] (Gateway reference 10106). London, HMSO.

Department of Health (2009a) *Implementing the next stage review revisions: The quality and productivity of challenge.* Letter from David Nicholson to all chief executives of primary care trusts, NHS trusts and foundation trusts in England (Gateway reference 12396). HMSO, London.

Department of Health (2009b) *Inspiring leaders: Leadership for quality.* HMSO, London.

De Salvo, L. (1999) *Writing as healing: How telling stories transforms our lives.* The Women's Press, London.

Dewey, J. (1933) *How we think.* JC Heath, Boston, MA.

Dickson, A. (1982) *A woman in your own right.* Quartet Books Limited, London.

Duffin, C. and Lipley, N. (2005) Fulfilling their potential? *Nursing Management,* 11(9): 7.

Farrell G. A. (2001) From tall poppies to squashed weeds: Why don't nurses pull together more? *Journal of Advanced Nursing,* 35: 26–33.

Faugier, J. and Woolnough, H. (2003) Lessons from LEO: Part two. *Nursing Management,* 10(3): 22–24.

Fay, B. (1987) *Critical social science.* Polity Press, Cambridge.

Ford, J. D., Ford, L. W. and D'melio, A. (2008) Resistance to change: The rest of the story. *Academy of Management Review,* 33(2): 362–77.

Foucault, M. (1979) *Discipline and punish: The birth of the prison* (trans. A. Sheridan). Vintage/Random House, New York.

Frank, A. (2002) *At the will of the body: Reflections on illness.* Mariner Books, New York.

Freemantle, D. (1992) *Incredible bosses.* McGraw Hill, Maidenhead.

Freidson, E. (1970) *Professional domination.* Aldine Atherton, Chicago, IL.

Freire, P. (1972) *Pedagogy of the oppressed.* Penguin Books, London.

French, J. R. P. and Raven, B. (1968) Bases of social power. In Cartright, D. (Ed.) *Studies in social power.* Institute of Social Research, Ann Arbor, MI.

Gaebler, T. and Osbourne, D. (1992) *Reinventing government.* Addison-Wesley, Reading, MA.

George A. Smathers Libraries (2005) *Guide to the Isabel Briggs Myers Papers 1885–1992 developed by the staff.* (Bulk dates: 1940–1980) Ms. Group 64 79.5 ln/ft (123 boxes). Online. Available from http://web.uflib.ufl.edu/spec/manauscript/guides/Myers.htm (Accessed June 2005).

George, B. (2003) *Authentic leadership.* Jossey-Bass, San Francisco, CA.

Gibran, K. (1926) *The prophet.* Heinemann, London.

Gibson, C. (1991) A concept analysis of empowerment. *Journal of Advanced Nursing,* 16: 354–61.

Gilley, K. (1997) *Leading from the heart.* Butterworth-Heinemann, Boston, MA.

Gilligan, C. (1982) *In a different voice.* Harvard University Press, Cambridge, MA.

Glouberman, D. (2003) *The joy of burnout.* Hodder & Stoughton, London.

Goldstein, J. (2002) *One dharma.* Rider, London.

Goleman, D., Boyatzis, R. and Mckee, A. (2002) *Primal leadership: Realizing the power of emotional intelligence.* Harvard Business School Press, Boston, MA.

Grant, A. and Greene, J. (2001) *Coach yourself: Make real change to your life.* Momentum Books, London.

Greenleaf, R. (2002) [1977] *Servant leadership: A journey into the nature of legitimate power and greatness.* Paulist Press, New York/Mahwah, NJ.

Hall, L. (1964) Nursing – what is it? *Canadian Nurse,* 60(2): 150–4.

Hawkins, D. (2002) *Power vs. force: The hidden determinants of human behaviour* (Revised edition). Hay House Inc., Carlsbad, CA.

Hawkins, P. and Shohet, R. (1989) *Supervision for the helping professions.* Open University Press, Buckingham.

Heidegger, M. (1962) *Being and time.* Basil Blackwell, Oxford.

Hersey, P. and Blanchard, K. (1982) *Management of organizational behaviour: Utilizing human resources* (4th edition). Prentice Hall, Englewood Cliffs, NJ.

Holyoake, D. D. (2000) Using transactional analysis to understand the supervisory process. *Nursing Standard,* 14(33): 37–41.

Honey, P. (2002) *Problem people: How to manage them.* Chartered Institute of Personnel and Development, London.

Honey, P. and Mumford, A. (1989) *The manual of learning styles.* Peter Money, Maidenhead.

Hooks, B. (1994) *Teaching to transgress: Education as the practice of freedom.* Routledge, New York.

Houle, C. O. (1961) *The inquiring mind.* University of Wisconsin Press, Madison, WI.

Humphris, D. (2002) Certainty in an uncertain world: The road ahead. *Nursing Management,* 9(2): 6–10.

James, O. (2003) *They f*** you up.* Bloomsbury Publishing, London.

Jaworski, J. (1998) *Synchronicity: The inner path of leadership.* Berrett-Koehler Publishers, San Francisco, CA.

Johns, C. (1990a) Setting standards: Self-medication. *Nursing Times,* 86(11): 40–1.

Johns, C. (1990b) Autonomy of primary nurses: The need to both facilitate and limit autonomy. *Journal of Advanced Nursing,* 15: 886–94.

Johns, C. (1992) Ownership and the harmonious team: Barriers to developing the therapeutic nursing team in primary nursing. *Journal of Clinical Nursing,* 1: 89–94.

Johns, C. (1996) *The Burford NDU model: Caring in practice.* Blackwell Science, Oxford.

Johns, C. (2001) Depending on the intent and emphasis of the supervisor, clinical supervision can be a different experience. *Journal of Nursing Management,* 9: 139–45.

Johns, C. (2003) Clinical supervision as a model for clinical leadership. *Journal of Nursing Management,* 11: 25–34.

Johns, C. (2004a) *Becoming a reflective practitioner* (2nd edition). Blackwell Publishing, Oxford.

Johns, C. (2004b) Balancing the winds. *Reflective Practice,* 5(3): 67–84.

Johns, C. (2009) *Becoming a reflective practitioner* (3rd edition). Wiley-Blackwell, Oxford.

Johns, C. (2010) (Ed.) *Guided reflection: A narrative approach to advancing practice* (2nd edition). Wiley-Blackwell, Oxford.

Johns, C. (2013) *Becoming a reflective practitioner* (4th edition). Wiley-Blackwell, Oxford.

Johns, C. (2014) People are not numbers to crunch. *British Journal of Cardiac Nursing,* 8(10): 466.

Jones, R. and Jones, G. (1996) *Earth dance drum*. Commune-A-Key Publishing, Salt Lake City, UT.

Kabat-Zin, J. (1994) *Wherever you go there you are*. Hyperion, New York.

Kerfoot, K. (2002) Leading the leaders: The challenge of leading an empowered organisation. *Dermatology Nursing*, 14(4): 273–5.

Kirkham, M. (1999) The culture of midwifery in the National Health Service in England. *Journal of Advanced Nursing*, 30(3): 732–39.

Kitching, D. (1993) Nursing leadership – myth or reality? *Journal of Nursing Management*, 1: 253–7.

Klein, D. (1976) Some notes on the dynamics of resistance to change: The defender role. In Bennis, W. G., Benne, K. D., Chin, R. and Corey, K. E. (Eds) *The planning of change* (3rd edition) Holt, Rinehart & Winston, New York, pp. 117–24.

Lather, P. (1993) Fertile obsession: Validity after post-structuralism. *The Sociological Quarterly*, 34: 673–93.

Latimer, J. (1995) The nursing process re-examined: Enrolment and translation. *Journal of Advanced Nursing*, 22: 213–30.

Levine, S. (1988) *Who dies? An investigation of conscious living and conscious dying*. Gateway Books, Bath.

Lewin, K. (1935) *A dynamic theory of personality*. McGraw-Hill, New York.

Lewin, K. (1951) *Field theory in social science*. Harper & Row, New York.

Lewin, K. cited in Schein, E. (1999) *Kurt Lewin's change theory in the field and in the classroom: Notes towards a model of managed learning* (online). Available from www.learning.mit.edu/res/wp/10006.html. (Accessed 5 January 2005).

Lewis, M. and Urmston, J. (2000) Flogging the dead horse: The myth of nursing empowerment? *Journal of Nursing Management*, 8: 209–13.

Liehr, P. (1989) A loving center: The core of true presence. *Nursing Science Quarterly*, 2(1): 7–8.

Lindberg, B., Zimmerman, B. and Plesek P. (1998) *Edgeware: Insights from complexity science for health care leaders*. VHA Press, Irving, TX.

Loori, J. Daido (2004) *The Zen of creativity: Cultivating your artistic life*. Ballantine Books, New York.

Manthey, M. (1980) *The practice of primary nursing*. Creative Nursing Management, Minneapolis, MN.

Marris, P. (1986) *Loss and change* (3rd edition). Routledge, London.

Marquis, B. L. and Huston, C. J. (1996) *Leadership roles and management functions in nursing* (2nd edition). Lippincott, Philadelphia, PA.

Mattingley, C. (1998) *Healing dramas and clinical plots: The narrative structure of experience*. Cambridge University Press, Cambridge.

Mayeroff, M. (1971) *On caring*. Harper Perennial, New York.

Mintzberg, H. (1973) *The nature of managerial work*. Harper & Row, New York.

Muir Gray, J. (1997) *Evidence-based health care: How to make health policy and management decisions*. Churchill Livingstone, New York.

Mycek, S. (1999) Teetering on the edge of chaos. *Trustee*, April: 10–13.

Navone, J. (1977) *Towards a theology of story*. St Paul Publications, Slough.

Northouse, P. (2001) *Leadership theory and practice* (2nd edition). Sage, Thousand Oaks, CA.

Oberle, K. (1991) A decade of research in locus of control: What have we learned? *Journal of Advanced Nursing*, 16: 800–6.

Okri, B. (1997) *A way of being free*. Phoenix House, London.

Olofsson, B., Bengtsson, C. and Brink, E. (2003) Absence of response: A study of nurses' experiences of stress in the workplace. *Journal of Nursing Management*, 11: 351–8.

Osho (1994) *No water no moon*. Elemental Books, Shaftesbury.

Ottaway, R. (1976) A change strategy to implement new norms, new styles and new environment in the work organization. *Personnel Review*, 5(1): 13–18.

Paley, J. (2002) Caring as a slave morality: Nietzchean themes in nursing ethics. *Journal of Advanced Nursing*, 40(1): 25–35.

Paramananda (2001) *A Deeper Beauty*. Windhorse Publications, Birmingham.

Pearson, A. (1983) *The clinical nursing unit*. Heinemann Medical Books, London.

Peck, M. (1978) *The road less travelled*. Rider, London.

Pinar, W. (1981) Whole, bright, deep with understanding: Issues in qualitative research and autobiographical method. *Journal of Curriculum Studies*, 13(3): 173–88.

Pirsig, R. (1974) *Zen and the art of motorcycle maintenance*. Vintage, London.

Porter-O'Grady, T. (1992) Transformational leadership in an age of chaos. *Nursing Administration Quarterly*, 17(1): 17–24.

Pratt, J., Gordon, P. and Plamping, D. (1999) *Working whole systems: Putting theory into practice in organisations*. The Kings Fund, London.

Prosser, S. (2010) *Servant leadership: More philosophy, less theory*. The Greenleaf Center for Servant Leadership, Westfield, IN.

Rael, J. (1993) *Being and vibration*. Council Oak Books, Tulsa, OK.

Remen, R. (2000) *My grandfather's blessings: Stories of strength, refuge and belonging*. Riverhead Books, New York.

Rinpoche, S. (1992) *The Tibetan book of living and dying*. Rider, London.

Rippon, S. (2001) Clinical leadership embracing a bold new agenda. *Nursing Management*, 8(6): 6–9.

Roberts, S. J. (1983) Oppressed group behaviour: Implications for nursing. *Advances in Nursing Science*, July: 21–30.

Roberts, S. J. (2000) Development of a positive professional identity: Liberating oneself from the oppressor within. *Advances in Nursing Science*, 22(4): 71–82.

Rodriguez, L. (1995) Selecting, developing, empowering and coaching staff. In Wise, Y. (Ed.) *Leading and Managing in Nursing*. C. V. Mosby, St. Louis, MS.

Rogers, A. (1998) Adult students – who are they? In Downie, C. M. and Basford, P. (Eds) *Teaching and assessing in clinical practice*. University of Greenwich, London.

Rosener, J. B. (1990) Ways women lead. *Harvard Business Review*, 68(6): 119–25.

Sacks, O. (1990) *Awakenings*. Picador, London.

Salzberg, S. (2002) *Faith: Trusting your own deepest experience*. Riverhead Books, New York.

Sangharakshita, B. (1988) *Know your mind: The psychological dimension of ethics in Buddhism*. Windhorse, Birmingham.

Schön, D. (1983) *The reflective practitioner*. Avebury, Aldershot.

Schön, D. (1987) *Educating the reflective practitioner*. Jossey-Bass, San Francisco, CA.

Schuster, J. P. (1994) Transforming your leadership style, *Association Management*, 46(1): 39–42.

Senge, P. M. (1990) *The fifth discipline. The art and practice of the learning organisation*. Doubleday/Currency, New York.

Sheehan, J. (1990) Investigating change in a nursing context. *Journal of Advanced Nursing*, 15: 81924.

Simon, R. and Dippo, D. (1986) On critical ethnographic work. *Anthropology and Education Quarterly*, 17: 195–202.

Skjorshammer, M. (2002) Understanding conflicts between health professionals: A narrative approach. *Qualitative Health Research,* 12: 915.

Sofarelli, D. and Brown, D. (1998) The need for nursing leadership in uncertain times. *Journal of Nursing Management*, 6, 201–7.

Stein, L. (1967) The doctor–nurse game. *Archives of General Psychiatry,* 16: 699–703.

Stewart, I. and Joines, V. (1987) *TA today: A new introduction to transactional analysis.* Russell Press, Nottingham.

Stokes, G. (1992) *On being old. The psychology of later life.* Falmer Press, London.

Susuki, S. (1999) *Zen mind, beginner's mind* (1st revised edition). Weatherhill, New York.

Swensen, S., Pugh, M., McMullan, C. and Kabcenell, A. (2013). *High-impact leadership: Improve care, improve the health of populations, and reduce costs.* IHI White Paper, Institute for Healthcare Improvement, Cambridge, MA. Online. Available at ihi.org.

Thomas, K. and Kilmann, R. (1974) *Thomas Kilmann Conflict Mode Instrument.* Xicom, Toledo, OH.

Tones, K. and Tilford, S. (1994) *Health education – Effectiveness, efficiency and equity.* Chapman & Hall, London.

Torbert, W. R. (1978) Educating toward shared purpose, self-direction and quality work. *Journal of Higher Education,* 49(2): 109–35.

Trofino, J. (1995) Transformational leadership in health care. *Nursing Management,* 26(8): 42–7.

Tschudin, V. (1999) Nurses matter: Reclaiming our professional identity. Macmillan Press, Basingstoke.

Tufnell, M. and Crickmay, C. (2004) *A widening field: Journeys in body and imagination.* Dance Books, Alton.

Tzu, L. (1999) *Tao Te Ching* (trans. Stephen Mitchell). Frances Lincoln, London.

Vail, P. (1996) *Learning as a way of being: Strategies for survival in a world of permanent white water.* Jossey-Bass, San Francisco, CA.

Valentine, P. (1994) Management of conflict: Do Women Handle It Differently? *Journal of Advanced Nursing*, 22: 142–49.

Wallerstein, N. and Bernstein, E. (1988) Empowerment education: Freire's ideas adapted to health education. *Health Education Quarterly,* 15: 379–94.

Watson, R. and Thompson, D. (2003) Will modern matrons carry on regardless? *Journal of Nursing Management,* 11: 65–8.

Webster, G. V. (1917) *Concerning osteopathy.* The Journal Printing Co., Kirksville, MO.

Wedderburn Tate, C. (1999) *Leadership in Nursing.* Churchill Livingstone, London.

West, M., Eckert, R., Steward, K. and Pasmore, B. (2014) *Developing collective leadership for health care.* King's Fund/Center for Creative Leadership, London.

Wheatley, M. J. (1999) *Leadership and the new science.* Berrett-Koehler Publishers, San Francisco, CA.

Wheatley, M. J. and Kellner-Rogers, M. (1996) *A simpler way.* Berrett-Koehler Publisher, San Francisco, CA.

Whetten, D., Cameron, K. and Woods, M. (1996) *Effective conflict management.* Harper Collins, London.

Wilber, K. (2001) *The eye of spirit.* Shambhala Publications, Boston, MA.

Wilkin, D., Gillam, S. and Coleman, A. (2001). *The national tracker survey of primary care groups and trusts 2000/2001: Modernising the NHS?* The National Primary Care Research and Development Centre, University of Manchester, Manchester.

Wilkinson, J. M. (1996) *Nursing process: A critical thinking approach.* Addison-Wesley, London.

Woolf, V. (1945) [1928] *A room of one's own.* Penguin Books, London.

Wuest, J. (1998) Setting boundaries: A strategy for precarious ordering of women's caring demands. *Research in Nursing and Health,* 21: 39–49.

Index